QUALITY THROUGH COLLABORATION

THE FUTURE OF RURAL HEALTH

Committee on the Future of Rural Health Care

Board on Health Care Services

INSTITUTE OF MEDICINE
OF THE NATIONAL ACADEMIES

THE NATIONAL ACADEMIES PRESS
Washington, D.C.
www.nap.edu

THE NATIONAL ACADEMIES PRESS • 500 Fifth Street, N.W. • Washington, DC 20001

NOTICE: The project that is the subject of this report was approved by the Governing Board of the National Research Council, whose members are drawn from the councils of the National Academy of Sciences, the National Academy of Engineering, and the Institute of Medicine. The members of the committee responsible for the report were chosen for their special competences and with regard for appropriate balance.

This study was supported by Contract No. 282-99-0045, T.O. #14 between the National Academy of Sciences and the Health Resources and Services Administration and the Agency for Healthcare and Research Quality. Support was also provided by Contract No. 03M00025301D from the Substance Abuse and Mental Health Services Agency and Contract No. P0105938 from the W. K. Kellogg Foundation. Any opinions, findings, conclusions, or recommendations expressed in this publication are those of the author(s) and do not necessarily reflect the views of the organizations or agencies that provided support for the project.

Library of Congress Cataloging-in-Publication Data

Quality through collaboration : the future of rural health / Committee on the Future of Rural Health Care, Board on Health Care Services.
   p. ; cm.
Includes bibliographical references and index.
ISBN 0-309-09439-9 (hardcover)
1. Rural health—United States. 2. Rural health services—United States.
[DNLM: 1. Rural Health Services—trends—United States. 2. Delivery of Health Care, Integrated—trends—United States. 3. Health Policy—United States. 4. Quality of Health Care—trends—United States.] I. Institute of Medicine (U.S.). Committee on the Future of Rural Health Care.
RA771.5.Q34 2005
362.1′04257—dc22

                    2004028192

Additional copies of this report are available from the National Academies Press, 500 Fifth Street, N.W., Lockbox 285, Washington, DC 20055; (800) 624-6242 or (202) 334-3313 (in the Washington metropolitan area); Internet, http://www.nap.edu.

For more information about the Institute of Medicine, visit the IOM home page at: **www.iom.edu**.

The serpent has been a symbol of long life, healing, and knowledge among almost all cultures and religions since the beginning of recorded history. The serpent adopted as a logotype by the Institute of Medicine is a relief carving from ancient Greece, now held by the Staatliche Museum in Berlin.

Cover photos reprinted with permission: (1) Town of Clear Lake, Iowa, copyright 2002 Roger F. Bindl; (2) Aquilla Walker, PharmD, Manatee County Rural Health Services, Inc., copyright 2004 University of South Florida AHEC; (3) Tomah Memorial Hospital, copyright 2004 Tomah Memorial Hospital; (4) Home Health Care Nurse, copyright 2004 Jeff Joiner; (5) A Rural Ambulance Nissan 4WD near Bright, Victoria, copyright 2004 Driver Improvement Consultancy Pty Ltd.; (6) UCL Telemedicine Program, copyright 1999 University College London. Other photos available publicly: (1) Performing Breathing Test, Indian Health Service Photo Gallery, Image #206; (2) Small Farms, Agricultural Research Service, Image #K8502-1; (3) Child Being Examined by Physicians, National Institute of Allergy and Infectious Disease.

"Knowing is not enough; we must apply.
Willing is not enough; we must do."
—Goethe

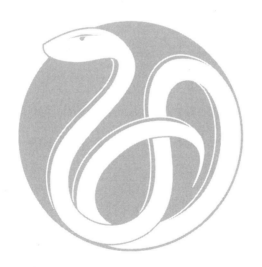

INSTITUTE OF MEDICINE
OF THE NATIONAL ACADEMIES

Adviser to the Nation to Improve Health

THE NATIONAL ACADEMIES
Advisers to the Nation on Science, Engineering, and Medicine

The **National Academy of Sciences** is a private, nonprofit, self-perpetuating society of distinguished scholars engaged in scientific and engineering research, dedicated to the furtherance of science and technology and to their use for the general welfare. Upon the authority of the charter granted to it by the Congress in 1863, the Academy has a mandate that requires it to advise the federal government on scientific and technical matters. Dr. Bruce M. Alberts is president of the National Academy of Sciences.

The **National Academy of Engineering** was established in 1964, under the charter of the National Academy of Sciences, as a parallel organization of outstanding engineers. It is autonomous in its administration and in the selection of its members, sharing with the National Academy of Sciences the responsibility for advising the federal government. The National Academy of Engineering also sponsors engineering programs aimed at meeting national needs, encourages education and research, and recognizes the superior achievements of engineers. Dr. Wm. A. Wulf is president of the National Academy of Engineering.

The **Institute of Medicine** was established in 1970 by the National Academy of Sciences to secure the services of eminent members of appropriate professions in the examination of policy matters pertaining to the health of the public. The Institute acts under the responsibility given to the National Academy of Sciences by its congressional charter to be an adviser to the federal government and, upon its own initiative, to identify issues of medical care, research, and education. Dr. Harvey V. Fineberg is president of the Institute of Medicine.

The **National Research Council** was organized by the National Academy of Sciences in 1916 to associate the broad community of science and technology with the Academy's purposes of furthering knowledge and advising the federal government. Functioning in accordance with general policies determined by the Academy, the Council has become the principal operating agency of both the National Academy of Sciences and the National Academy of Engineering in providing services to the government, the public, and the scientific and engineering communities. The Council is administered jointly by both Academies and the Institute of Medicine. Dr. Bruce M. Alberts and Dr. Wm. A. Wulf are chair and vice chair, respectively, of the National Research Council.

www.national-academies.org

COMMITTEE ON THE FUTURE OF RURAL HEALTH CARE

Study Staff

JANET CORRIGAN, Senior Board Director
PHILIP ASPDEN, Senior Program Officer
LYNNE PAGE SNYDER, Program Officer
JULIE WOLCOTT, Program Officer
GOOLOO WUNDERLICH,* Senior Program Officer
BINA RUSSELL, Senior Project Assistant

Editorial Consultants

RONA BRIERE, Briere Associates, Inc.
ALISA DECATUR, Briere Associates, Inc.

Content Consultants

DAVID A. KINDIG, Emeritus Professor of Population Health Sciences, University of Wisconsin Medical School

---

*Served until February 2003

Reviewers

This report has been reviewed in draft form by individuals chosen for their diverse perspectives and technical expertise, in accordance with procedures approved by the NRC Report Review Committee. The purpose of this independent review is to provide candid and critical comments that will assist the institution in making its published report as sound as possible and to ensure that the report meets institutional standards for objectivity, evidence, and responsiveness to the study charge. The review comments and draft manuscript remain confidential to protect the integrity of the deliberative process. We wish to thank the following individuals for their review of this report:

KIM BATEMAN, HealthInsight
LONNIE R. BRISTOW, Past-President, American Medical Association
PATRICIA LASKY, School of Nursing, University of Wisconsin-Madison
JAMES A. MERCHANT, College of Public Health, University of Iowa
KEITH MUELLER, Center for Rural Health Policy Analysis, University of Nebraska Medical Center
ELAINE POWER, National Quality Forum
KAREN RHEUBAN, Office of Continuing Medical Education, University of Virginia
SALLY K. RICHARDSON, West Virginia Institute for Health Policy Research, West Virginia University

JOHN R. WHEAT, College of Community Health Sciences, University of Alabama

Although the reviewers listed above have provided many constructive comments and suggestions, they were not asked to endorse the conclusions or recommendations nor did they see the final draft of the report before its release. The review of this report was overseen by **Neal A. Vanselow, Chancellor Emeritus, Tulane University Health Sciences Center,** and **Charles E. Phelps, University of Rochester.** Appointed by the National Research Council and Institute of Medicine, they were responsible for making certain that an independent examination of this report was carried out in accordance with institutional procedures and that all review comments were carefully considered. Responsibility for the final content of this report rests entirely with the authoring committee and the institution.

Preface

In too many ways, rural communities have been at the margins of the health care quality movement. Most quality initiatives in the United States have been developed with urban health care features in mind and as a result have not always been directly applicable to rural health care settings. Before formulating a health care quality agenda in rural America, it will be necessary to determine the rural relevance of quality efforts broadly, while also developing new quality initiatives that directly recognize distinctive features of both the context in which care is given and care systems themselves in rural settings. For example, inpatient care in rural hospitals is often a smaller part of the total set of services than is the case in urban hospitals. Smaller case volumes and long-standing shortages of key health care services, such as those for mental health and substance abuse, draw a mix of providers different from the norm in urban settings. Historically, moreover, the financing of rural health care has been a particularly fragile endeavor. Along with the lack of established applicability of many quality efforts to rural settings, access and finance concerns have frequently hampered the ability of rural health care providers to fully address quality improvement.

While acknowledging these challenges, the Institute of Medicine's (IOM) Committee on the Future of Rural Health Care has charted an agenda for rural communities that fulfills the six aims set forth in the 2001 IOM report *Crossing the Quality Chasm: A New Health System for the 21st Cen-*

tury of making health care safe, effective, patient-centered, timely, efficient, and equitable. This agenda also reflects the need to improve both the quality of personal health care and the health of the rural population as a whole, as well as to apply the newest tools available, such as information technology, to the work of delivering high-quality health care in rural settings. Specifically, the agenda addresses the need to modify existing quality indicators and processes to reflect the special characteristics of rural communities, to strengthen the human resources for health care networks in rural areas, and to implement a health care information infrastructure across rural communities. In the process, the committee also notes the importance of leveraging the unique strengths of rural communities.

Implementation of the recommendations contained in this report, combined with the determination of rural communities to develop creative ways of improving their own health care systems, will set the stage for the consistent delivery of high-quality health care regardless of where one lives in the United States. Capitalizing on their unique strengths, rural communities and health care systems can meet the expectations associated with delivering the highest quality of care possible.

Finally, this report represents the culmination of the dedicated efforts of many individuals. I would like to thank my fellow committee members, who worked long and diligently on this challenging study; the many experts who provided formal testimony to the committee and informal advice throughout the study; and the staff of the Health Care Services Board who managed the study and coordinated the writing of the final report.

Mary Wakefield, Ph.D., R.N., F.A.A.N.
Chair
November 2004

Foreword

The Institute of Medicine (IOM) has had a long-standing focus on quality of care. In the first phase of the IOM quality initiative, the National Roundtable on Health Care Quality highlighted serious problems with the overall quality of care delivered in the United States. In the second phase, two reports, *To Err Is Human: Building a Safer Health System* and *Crossing the Quality Chasm: A New Health System for the 21st Century*, were released. Both reports called for a fundamental redesign of the health care delivery system.

In the third and current phase, the IOM has sought to elaborate and to realize the vision of a future health system as set forth in the *Quality Chasm* report. The *Quality Chasm* report identified six aims for the delivery of health care: care should be safe, effective, patient-centered, timely, efficient, and equitable. Among the profound changes needed to achieve these aims are that information technology must play a central role in support of the delivery of care; that provider payment systems must reward the provision of quality care; and that the education and training of health professionals must encompass evidence-based skills and working in interdisciplinary teams.

The study presented here marks another step in this third phase of the IOM's quality initiative. Rural America, with about a fifth of the U.S. population, is a vibrant part of the nation. Its people are independent-minded, but with a strong sense of the need to work with others to provide services that many urban dwellers take for granted. Rural communities differ widely, both among themselves and from urban communities, in their economic and social characteristics. They also vary greatly in their population densities and their remoteness from urban areas. The set of health problems faced by rural communities differs from those faced by urban communities. Thus, realizing the vision and six aims set forth in the *Quality Chasm* report poses special challenges for rural areas that are not present in urban areas.

The present report identifies ways to assure that rural America benefits from the many changes unfolding in the health care sector and especially from efforts to redesign health care to deliver the highest possible quality.

Harvey V. Fineberg, M.D., Ph.D.
President, Institute of Medicine
November 2004

Acknowledgments

The Committee on the Future of Rural Health Care wishes to acknowledge the many people whose contributions and support made this report possible.

The committee benefited from presentations by a number of experts on various issues addressed during its meetings over the past 14 months. The following individuals shared their research, experience, and perspectives with the committee: Michael Beachler, Pennsylvania State University; Marcia Brand, Health Resources and Services Administration (HRSA); Kathleen Buckwalter, University of Iowa; Helen Burstin, Agency for Healthcare Research and Quality (AHRQ); Carolyn Clancy, AHRQ; Elizabeth Duke, HRSA; Robert Galvin, General Electric Company; Larry Gamm, Texas A&M University; Stuart Guterman, Centers for Medicare and Medicaid Services; Brent James, InterMountain Health Care; David Kibbe, American Academy of Family Physicians; Ravi Nemana, The Health Technology Center; Richard Palagi, St. John's Lutheran Hospital; Cathleen Pfaff, Cypress Healthcare, LLC; Steven Pierdon, Geisinger Health Systems; Howard Rabinowitz, Thomas Jefferson University; Regina Schofield, Office of the Secretary, Department of Health and Human Services (DHHS); Ulonda Shamwell, Substance Abuse and Mental Health Services Agency (SAMHSA); Glenn Steele, Geisinger Health Systems; Walter Stewart, Geisinger Health Systems; and Pamela Wirth, Susquehanna Health System.

A number of experts were important sources of information, generously contributing their time and knowledge to further the committee's aims. Sunga Kay Carter, Research Coordinator at the Emergency Medical Services for Children National Resource Center, provided useful unpublished research data on workforce strength in emergency medical services. The committee also thanks David E. Cockley, Assistant Professor, Department of Health Sciences, James Madison University; Jeptha W. Dalston, President and CEO, Accrediting Commission on Education for Health Services Administration; Peter Keller, Professor and Chairperson, Department of Psychology, Mansfield University; and Liane Pinero Kluge, Association of University Programs in Health Administration.

The committee commissioned four papers that provided important background information and insights for the report. Calvin Beale, in association with John Cromartie, U.S. Department of Agriculture, authored a paper describing and analyzing data needed to understand rural population trends, the changes and diversity in the rural population, and the issues associated with defining "rural." Larry Gamm, in collaboration with Linnae Hutchinson, Texas A&M University, produced a paper describing and analyzing prevalence and rural disparities in mental health conditions and substance abuse behaviors, along with barriers to accessing professionals and services in these areas. Keith Mueller, in association with Timothy D. McBride, University of Nebraska Medical Center, authored a paper describing and analyzing reimbursement, financing, and payment policies for rural health care. Thomas Nesbitt, working with Peter Yellowlees, University of California-Davis Health System, wrote a paper on information technology for the rural health care context.

The committee also benefited from the work of other committees and staff of the Institute of Medicine that conducted studies relevant to this report. The committee benefited particularly from the work of the Committee on the Quality of Health Care in America and the Committee on Identifying Priority Areas for Quality Improvement. The committee on the Quality of Health Care in America produced the 2000 report *To Err Is Human: Building a Safer Health System* and the 2001 report *Crossing the Quality Chasm: A New Health System for the 21st Century*. The committee on Identifying Priority Areas for Quality Improvement produced the 2003 report *Priority Areas for National Action: Transforming Health Care Quality*.

The committee recognizes the hard work of staff at the Institute of Medicine. Maria Hewitt of the National Cancer Policy Board, Institute of Medicine, was very gracious in lending copies of a study on rural health and rural emergency medical services, conducted from 1989 to 1990 during her tenure at the Office of Technology Assessment.

Finally, funding for this project came from HRSA, AHRQ, SAMHSA, and the W. K. Kellogg Foundation. The committee extends special thanks to HRSA, AHRQ, SAMHSA, and Kellogg for providing this support.

Contents

Executive Summary

Rural America is a vital component of American society. Representing nearly 20 percent of the population, rural communities, like urban landscapes, are rich in cultural diversity. From the Native American Indian tribes and Hispanic communities of the southwest, to the African American communities of the Mississippi Bayou, to the Amish settlements of Pennsylvania, to the European descendants of the Great Plains, rural communities are home to many of the earliest Americans, as well as more recent immigrants.

Rural communities are heterogeneous in other ways as well, differing in population density, remoteness from urban areas, and economic and social characteristics. Many such communities adjacent to urban areas are growing in population as they become popular destinations for those willing to commute or telecommute to jobs in urban areas. Rural America also includes thinly settled frontier areas, many with stagnant or declining economies as the result of an inability to transition from what was once a largely agricultural settlement.

In general, the smaller, poorer, and more isolated a rural community is, the more difficult it is to ensure the availability of high-quality health services. Compared with urban communities, rural communities tend to have fewer health care organizations and professionals of all types, less choice and competition among them, and broad variation in their availability at the local level.

THE HEALTH CARE QUALITY CHALLENGE

In 2001, the Institute of Medicine (IOM) released the report *Crossing the Quality Chasm: A New Health System for the 21st Century.* Based on a large body of evidence documenting serious shortcomings in the American health care system overall, the IOM report calls for fundamental reform of the U.S. health care system. The report identifies six aims for quality improvement—health care should be safe, effective, patient-centered, timely, efficient, and equitable. Recognizing the magnitude of the changes required to address the quality challenge, the IOM launched the *Quality Chasm* series. Thus far, eight reports have been produced in this series, addressing various aspects of the agenda for change. This report on rural health care quality is a part of this series.

The IOM Committee on the Future of Rural Health Care was asked to

- Assess the quality of health care in rural areas.
- Develop a conceptual framework for a core set of services and the essential infrastructure necessary to deliver those services to rural communities.
- Recommend priority objectives, and identify changes in policies and programs required to achieve those objectives, including, but not limited to, payment policies and the necessary information and communications technology (ICT) infrastructure.
- Consider implications for federal programs and policy.

In many respects, rural communities have been on the periphery of discussions of national health care quality. A roadmap for applying the quality agenda now evolving at the national level to sparsely populated areas is needed.

ADDRESSING THE QUALITY CHALLENGE IN A RURAL CONTEXT

Rural communities likely face the same quality challenge as urban communities. Although the evidence pertaining specifically to rural areas is sparse, what does exist corroborates the general finding that, as documented for the nation overall in the *Quality Chasm* report, the level of quality falls far short of what it should be.

Some of the quality shortcomings in rural areas stem from the lack of access to "core health care services," defined for purposes of this report as primary care in the community, emergency medical services, hospital care, long-term care, mental health and substance abuse services, oral health care, and public health services. For some core health care services, most notably emergency medical services, mental health and substance abuse services, and oral health care, access is severely constrained in many if not most rural communities by long-standing shortages of qualified health professionals. Many rural communities have difficulty attracting and retaining clinicians because of concerns about isolation, limited health facilities, or a lack of employment and education opportunities for their families. Although steps have been taken in recent years to introduce a more favorable financial climate for rural health care providers, an underresourced health care delivery infrastructure persists.

Rural communities also confront a different mix of health and health care needs than do urban areas. Rural populations tend to be older than urban populations and to experience higher rates of limitations in daily activities as a result of chronic conditions. Rural populations exhibit poorer health behaviors (i.e., higher rates of smoking and obesity and lower rates of exercise) relative to most urban populations, although there is variability in health behaviors among rural communities. Unless action is taken now, the future burden of chronic disease in many rural communities will be enormous.

The IOM committee developed a five-pronged strategy to address the quality challenges in rural communities:

• Adopt an integrated, prioritized approach to addressing both personal and population health needs at the community level;
• Establish a stronger quality improvement support structure to assist rural health systems and professionals in acquiring knowledge and tools to improve quality;
• Enhance the human resource capacity of rural communities, including the education, training, and deployment of health care professionals, and the preparedness of rural residents to engage actively in improving their health and health care;
• Monitor rural health care systems to ensure that they are financially stable and provide assistance in securing the necessary capital for system redesign; and
• Invest in building an ICT infrastructure, which has enormous potential to enhance health and health care over the coming decades.

ADDRESSING PERSONAL AND POPULATION HEALTH NEEDS

In 1990, the IOM adopted the following definition of quality of care:

Quality of care is the degree to which health services for individuals and populations increase the likelihood of desired health outcomes and are consistent with current professional knowledge (IOM, 1990, p. 4).

The above definition is consistent with the view that the health care system of the twenty-first century should balance and integrate the need for personal health care with broader communitywide initiatives that target the entire population and the environment (IOM, 2003). Many factors influence the health of individuals and populations, including the environment, social behaviors, and genetic predispositions.

The committee encourages rural communities to build a population health focus into decision making within the health care sector, as well as in other key areas (e.g., education, community and environmental planning) that influence population health. For example, there are many effective interventions available to rural communities to reduce the health burden of diabetes, some best implemented through the personal health care delivery system (e.g., reminder systems to prompt patients and clinicians when annual eye and foot exams are due) and others through communitywide programs (e.g., public policies that favor the provision of more nutritious food in public eating establishments and schools). Making explicit the full range of options available to rural communities to improve personal and population health should lead to more optimal allocation of scarce financial resources. Future work is needed to identify and prioritize the interventions that are available to rural communities to improve health and health care.

Key Finding 1. A wide range of interventions are available to improve health and health care in rural America, but priorities for implementation are not yet clear. The Health Resources and Services Administration is the obvious agency to take the lead in setting priorities, in collaboration with other federal agencies, such as the Agency for Healthcare Research and Quality and the Centers for Disease Control and Prevention, as well as with rural stakeholders. This would entail systematically cataloguing and evaluating the potential interventions to improve health care quality and population health in rural communities.

Each rural community will then need to set priorities for addressing personal and population health needs, and develop and implement an action plan. An earlier IOM report, *Fostering Rapid Advances in Health Care: Learning from System Demonstrations,* recommends the conduct of a set of community-level demonstrations intended to produce the first generation of twenty-first-century community health systems focused on meeting personal and population health needs. This IOM committee endorses this "bottom-up" approach to health system reform, and believes that rural communities, because of their smaller scale and other unique characteristics, offer an excellent setting for undertaking rapid-cycle experimentation.

Recommendation 1. Congress should provide the appropriate authority and resources to the Department of Health and Human Services to support comprehensive health system reform demonstrations in five rural communities. These demonstrations should evaluate alternative models for achieving greater integration of personal and population health services and innovative approaches to the financing and delivery of health services, with the goal of meeting the six quality aims of the *Quality Chasm* report. The Agency for Healthcare Research and Quality, working collaboratively with the Health Resources and Services Administration, should ensure that the lessons learned from these demonstrations are disseminated to other communities, both urban and rural.

Strong leadership will be needed to achieve significant improvements in health and health care in rural communities. Comprehensive community-based efforts will require extensive collaboration, both between stakeholders within the health care sector, and between health care and other sectors. It will be necessary to mobilize all types of institutions (e.g., health care, educational, social, and faith-based) to both augment and support the contributions of health professionals.

Key Finding 2. Rural communities engaged in health system redesign would likely benefit from leadership training programs. Such training programs could be provided by the Agency for Healthcare Research and Quality and the Office of Rural Health Policy working collaboratively with private- and public-sector organizations involved in leadership development, such as the National Council for Healthcare Leadership and the W. K. Kellogg Foundation's Leadership for Community Change Program.

ESTABLISHING A QUALITY IMPROVEMENT SUPPORT STRUCTURE

To achieve the six quality aims, rural communities must establish comprehensive quality improvement programs. Since the release of the *Quality Chasm* report, a great deal of national and local attention has been focused on enhancing the health care sector's quality improvement capabilities. Because of their small scale and low operating margins, rural providers have found it difficult to make such investments.

Although many of the elements of an effective quality improvement infrastructure will be the same for rural and urban areas, some customization is needed for rural areas. For example, when care processes in rural and urban areas differ because of differences in the mix of available services (e.g., urban areas have more ready access to tertiary-level care), rural-specific comparative data on some aspects of the care process (e.g., emergency care, stabilization, and transfer services for acute myocardial infarction patients) are most useful for quality improvement purposes.

For the most part, current quality improvement programs and tools available at the national and local levels focus on the personal health care system. To assist rural communities in their efforts to promote both personal and population health, further thought should be given to how best to adapt quality improvement knowledge and tools (e.g., evidence-based reports, practice guidelines, standardized performance measure sets) to support an integrated approach to decision making. Rural communities must also have the flexibility and assistance needed to develop quality improvement programs likely to have the greatest impact in a rural context. In some areas, for example, a communitywide or even regional quality improvement program is likely to be preferable to having each provider setting develop its own approach. To this end, the Department of Health and Human Services needs to develop a coordinated and tailored approach to meeting the needs of rural communities.

> **Recommendation 2. The Department of Health and Human Services should establish a Rural Quality Initiative to coordinate and accelerate efforts to measure and improve the quality of personal and population health care programs in rural areas. This initiative should be coordinated by the Health Resources and Services Administration's Office of Rural Health Policy, with guidance from a Rural Quality Advisory Panel consisting of experts from the private sector and state and local governments having knowledge and experience in rural health care quality measurement and improvement.**

The agenda of this proposed initiative should include the following:

- *Applying evidence to practice*—The Agency for Healthcare Research and Quality should assume a lead role in developing educational programs and tools to assist rural communities in applying evidence to practice.
- *Standardized measure set for rural communities*—The Rural Quality Advisory Panel should work collaboratively with stakeholders from both the public and private sectors on the identification of appropriate standardized measures for rural areas, including: (1) measures from leading measure sets that are applicable to all geographic areas; (2) where necessary, new measures to reflect aspects of care processes that are rural-specific; and (3) standardized population health measures to be piloted in rural areas.
- *Public reporting*—Centers for Medicare and Medicaid Services (CMS) and the Rural Quality Advisory Panel should work collaboratively to ensure that rural providers are included in public reporting initiatives and that public reports for rural providers make fair and meaningful comparisons.
- *Community-based technical assistance*—CMS should ensure that the Quality Improvement Organizations devote resources to rural areas commensurate with the proportion of Medicare beneficiaries in a state that reside in rural areas. Consideration should be given to establishing a Quality Improvement Organization Support Center to focus on application of the above standardized quality measures to rural areas. The Office of Rural Health Policy should convene a series of regional conferences for Critical Access Hospitals, rural health clinics, community health centers, and other providers to share quality improvement processes and techniques.
- *Data repository*—CMS should expand its data repositories to include rural-specific quality data so that rural providers have access to both urban and rural data for benchmarking purposes.

STRENGTHENING HUMAN RESOURCES

Human resources are critical to every rural community's efforts to improve individual and population health. Human resources include health care professionals, both those in practice and those in training, as well as the population at large in the community.

The IOM committee believes that a renewed and vigorous effort must be made to enhance the health professions workforce in rural areas. This effort should focus on enhancing the quality improvement knowledge and skills of practicing professionals and the supply and preparedness of future professionals working in rural areas.

The 2003 IOM report *Health Professions Education: A Bridge to Quality* identifies five core competencies that all health care professionals should master to provide high-quality care: (1) provide patient-centered care, (2) work in interdisciplinary teams, (3) employ evidence-based practice, (4) apply quality improvement, and (5) utilize informatics. The federal government sponsors numerous workforce education programs that provide experientially based training for practicing health professionals, and these should be expanded to focus greater attention on helping professionals master the core competencies.

> **Recommendation 3. Congress should provide appropriate resources to the Health Resources and Services Administration to expand experientially based workforce training programs in rural areas to ensure that all health care professionals master the core competencies of providing patient-centered care, working in interdisciplinary teams, employing evidence-based practice, applying quality improvement, and utilizing informatics. These competencies are relevant to the many discipline-specific and multidisciplinary programs supported under Titles VII and VIII of the Social Security Act.**

Specifically, more stable and generous funding should be provided for the Quentin Burdick Program to conduct demonstrations in several rural communities that provide for (1) the training of leadership teams to mobilize community resources, (2) communitywide health literacy programs, and (3) interdisciplinary health professions education in the core competencies essential to improving quality. Workforce programs such as the Health Resources and Services Administration's (HRSA) funding of Area Health Education Centers, Health Education and Training Centers, and Geriatric Education Centers should explicitly target rural localities, and broaden their scope beyond physician supply to include midlevel providers in specialties in short supply in rural areas (e.g., mental health and substance abuse services and emergency care). Also, programs that recruit students from minority and underserved communities for health professions careers in rural areas—such as the Health Careers Opportunity Program, HRSA's Centers of Excellence program, scholarship and loan repayment programs for disadvantaged students, and such programs offered by the Indian Health Service—should expand their recruitment and placement efforts in rural communities.

In expanding experientially based workforce training programs, the federal government should place particular emphasis on the types of health professionals that are in very short supply and on the geographic areas experiencing the greatest difficulty in recruitment and retention. Essential health professions data at the state and local levels are needed to support decisions about targeting resources to rural areas, including the designation of shortage areas. This is especially true with regard to mental and behavioral health services and oral health.

Key Finding 3. To target workforce training programs most effectively, federal, state, and local governments need better information on the current supply and types of health professionals. Data that would be particularly useful include the numbers of providers and provider hours of clinical practice, practice specialties, and sites of service. Financial and policy incentives at the federal and state levels could be put in place to facilitate the gathering, analysis, and retention of health professions workforce data that are comparable across states.

Enhancing education and training programs for practicing professionals is an important first step, but it will not be enough. Fundamental change in health professions education programs and institutions will be needed to produce an adequate future supply of properly educated professionals for rural and frontier communities. A multifaceted approach to the recruitment and retention of health professionals in rural areas is needed, including interventions at every point along the rural workforce pipeline: (1) enhanced preparation of rural elementary and high school students to pursue health careers; (2) stronger commitment of health professions education programs to recruiting students from rural areas, educating and training students in those areas, and adopting rural-appropriate curricula; and (3) a variety of strong incentives for health professionals to seek and retain employment in rural communities.

Enhancements to the basic curriculum, particularly the science curriculum, for middle and high school students are needed to better prepare rural students for careers in the health professions. HRSA's Office of Rural Health Policy could work collaboratively with the various federal agencies (e.g., Bureau of Health Professions, Department of Education, Bureau of Indian Affairs, and Indian Health Service), professional associations, and rural constituencies to identify appropriate enhancements and develop an action plan. A rural health professions mentoring program might be established to expose rural students to potential careers in health care. Changes are also needed in health professions education programs.

Recommendation 4. Schools of medicine, dentistry, nursing, allied health, and public health and programs in mental and behavioral health should:

• Work collaboratively to establish outreach programs to rural areas to attract qualified applicants.
• Locate a meaningful portion of the educational experience in rural communities. Universities and 4-year colleges should expand distance learning programs and/or pursue formal arrangements with community and other colleges, including tribal and traditionally African American colleges, located in rural areas to extend the array of rural-based education options while encouraging students to pursue higher levels of education.
• Make greater effort to recruit faculty with experience in rural practice, and develop rural-relevant curricula addressing areas that are key to improving health and health care, including the five core competencies (i.e., providing patient-centered care, working in interdisciplinary teams, employing evidence-based practice, applying quality improvement, and utilizing informatics), the fundamentals of population health, and leadership skills.
• Develop rural training tracks and fellowships that (1) provide students with rotations in rural provider sites; (2) emphasize primary care practice; and (3) provide cross-training in key areas of shortage in rural communities, such as emergency and trauma care, mental health, and obstetrics.

Furthermore, the federal government should provide financial incentives for residency training programs to provide rural tracks by linking some portion of the graduate medical education payments under Medicare to achievement of this goal.

The residents of rural communities also have a key role to play in improving population health. Residents can contribute to improving their own health and that of others by pursuing healthy behaviors and complying with treatment regimens, assuming appropriate caregiving roles for family members and neighbors, and volunteering for community health improvement efforts. As is the case with many urban populations, many rural populations have low levels of health literacy (the degree to which individuals have the capacity to obtain, process, and understand basic health information) that currently hamper efforts to engage residents in health-related activities. The Department of Education and state education agencies should work in partnership with local nonprofit literacy associations and libraries to measure and improve the health literacy of rural residents by, among other things, providing access to Internet-based health resources.

PROVIDING ADEQUATE AND TARGETED FINANCIAL RESOURCES

To achieve the six quality aims, rural communities must have adequate and appropriately targeted financial resources. In the health care sector overall, a great deal of experimentation is currently under way to identify ways of better aligning payment incentives with the quality aims, and rural communities should be part of these efforts. At the same time, it is important to recognize that, historically, rural health care systems have been financially fragile, and many still have small operating margins, making it difficult for them to participate in innovative efforts intended to stimulate fundamental redesign of the delivery system.

Many public- and private-sector purchasers are conducting demonstrations or pilot projects that make some portion of provider payments contingent upon performance. The committee supports these early efforts to redesign payment programs and is concerned that rural communities may be left behind. It would be wise to conduct demonstration projects in rural communities to field test the applicability of both standardized performance measures and performance-based payment approaches to rural providers.

> **Recommendation 5. The Centers for Medicare and Medicaid Services should establish 5-year pay-for-performance demonstration projects in five rural communities starting in fiscal year 2006. During the first 18 months, the communities should receive grants and technical assistance for establishing processes to capture the patient data and other information needed to assess performance using a standardized performance measure set appropriate for rural communities. For the remaining 3.5 years, different approaches to implementing pay for performance should be tested in the various demonstration sites. The selected communities should be diverse with respect to socio-demographic variables, as well as the degree and type of formal integration of local and regional providers.**

The proposed demonstration projects will likely yield many important lessons learned. CMS could work collaboratively with HRSA to ensure that this information is widely disseminated to rural stakeholders, as well as to public and private purchasers engaged in pay-for-performance programs.

Recognizing that the health system is experiencing a period of fundamental change, careful attention should also be paid to ensuring the financial stability of rural health care delivery systems. Although significant steps have been taken to correct historical underpayment of rural providers under Medicare, the operating margins of many rural hospitals are still low, and concerns about the equity of physician payments persist. Rural providers have been heavily impacted as states have modified eligibility criteria or lowered provider payments under Medicaid and the Children's Health Insurance Program in response to worsening state financial conditions.

Recommendation 6. Rural health care delivery systems must be sufficiently stable financially to underwrite investments in human resources and information and communications technology and to implement pay-for-performance initiatives. The Agency for Healthcare Research and Quality should produce a report by no later than fiscal year 2006 analyzing the aggregate impact of changes in the Medicare program, state Medicaid programs, private health plans, and insurance coverage on the financial stability of rural health care providers. The report should detail specific actions that should be taken, if needed, to ensure sufficient financial stability for rural health care delivery systems to undertake the desired changes described in this report.

The IOM committee also wants to draw special attention to the very limited availability of mental health and substance abuse services in many rural communities, which is likely attributable in part to a lack of adequate funding. The committee recognizes that this is a complex area. The mental health needs of populations are diverse, and mental health care services are provided in both general and specialized settings and by a plethora of health care professionals. Patients likely have different preferences for settings and providers, and there may well be differences in the quality, accessibility, and cost of services by type of setting and provider. The financing of mental health services is equally complex, consisting of a patchwork of direct service programs financed through federal and state grants and public and private insurance programs.

Recommendation 7. The Health Resources and Services Administration and the Substance Abuse and Mental Health Services Administration should conduct a comprehensive assessment of the availability and quality of mental health and substance abuse services in rural

areas. This assessment should cover services provided in both primary care and specialty settings, and should include the following:

- A review of (1) the various insurance and direct service programs in the public and private sectors that provide financial support for the delivery of mental health and substance abuse services, and (2) the populations served by these payers and programs.
- An evaluation of the adequacy of current funding, and an analysis of alternative options for better aligning the various funding sources and programs to improve the accessibility and quality of these services. Attention should be focused on identifying and analyzing options designed to encourage collaboration between primary care and specialty settings.

UTILIZING INFORMATION AND COMMUNICATIONS TECHNOLOGY

ICT is a powerful tool with great potential to enhance health and health care in rural communities. Appropriate use of ICT can bridge distances by providing more immediate access to clinical knowledge, specialized expertise, and services not readily available in sparsely populated areas. However, many rural communities are unprepared to participate fully in the information age, having little or no access to the Internet and populations with minimal ICT experience. Most rural health care systems are in critical need of financial and technical assistance to establish electronic health records (EHRs) and secure platforms for health data exchange.

To ensure that no rural community is left behind as the nation moves to EHRs and an electronic highway for health data exchange, the committee has identified a strategy consisting of six action items: (1) including a rural component in the National Health Information Infrastructure (NHII) plan, (2) providing all rural communities with high-speed access to the Internet, (3) eliminating regulatory barriers to the use of telemedicine, (4) providing financial assistance to rural providers for investments in EHRs and ICT, (5) fostering ICT collaborations and demonstrations in rural areas, and (6) providing ongoing educational and technical assistance to rural communities so they can make the best use of ICT.

With the recent establishment of the Office of the National Coordinator for Health Information Technology, the federal government has assumed a leadership role in the development of the NHII over the next 10 years. If rural communities are to participate fully in the NHII, it is essential that the national planning process take into consideration the specific challenges faced by rural communities and target program activities and resources to meet these challenges.

Recommendation 8. The Office of the National Coordinator for Health Information Technology should incorporate a rural focus, including frontier areas, into its planning and developmental activities for the NHII.

• **The NHII strategic plan should include a component that is specific to rural and frontier areas, and this component should provide the programmatic and financial resources necessary for rural areas to participate fully in the NHII.**
• **The Office of Rural Health Policy should be designated as the lead agency for coordination of rural health input to the Office of the National Coordinator for Health Information Technology. In providing this input, the Office of Rural Health Policy should seek the expert advice of the Department of Health and Human Services' Rural Task Force.**

Many health-related ICT applications require access to high-speed Internet connections; however, broadband networks have not yet reached many rural and frontier communities. Broadband networks can benefit rural communities as a whole by giving local firms direct access to customers, suppliers, and larger markets, thus making it less expensive and more efficient for firms to locate in rural areas. In addition, these networks make it possible for residents of small towns to participate in distance education, training, and learning opportunities, a capability that is particularly important for building a health professions workforce and promoting health literacy.

Rural areas face another barrier to use of the Internet—the cost associated with the use of telecommunications lines. Surcharges and administrative fees levied by local area telecommunications access (LATA) networks often make data exchange prohibitively expensive, and this is especially true when the data transmission is between geographic areas located in different LATA networks.

Recommendation 9. Congress should take appropriate steps to ensure that rural communities are able to access and use the Internet for the full range of health-related applications. Specifically, consideration should be given to:

- Expanding and coordinating the efforts of federal agencies to extend broadband networks into rural areas.
- Prohibiting local area telecommunications access networks from imposing surcharges for the transfer of health messages across regions.
- Expanding the Universal Service Fund's Rural Health Care Program to allow the participation of all rural providers and to increase the amount of the subsidy.

The regulatory and payment environments have a significant impact on the ability of providers to make the best use of ICT. Currently, the use of telemedicine and other ICT applications is impeded by the absence of clear and consistent definitions and requirements across (1) state governments that license health professionals; (2) health care organizations (e.g., hospitals, health plans, nursing homes) that credential clinicians for practice within the organization; and (3) major payers, such as Medicare, that establish payment policies for telemedicine services.

Key Finding 4. Telehealth warrants special attention to facilitate its use while maintaining appropriate regulatory protections. Some changes in government regulatory processes and health insurance programs may be desirable, but a detailed analysis of current practices for purposes of identifying barriers to telehealth has yet to be conducted. The Office of the National Coordinator for Health Information Technology might provide leadership and coordination for such work.

If rural communities are to benefit from the NHII, financial assistance from the federal government will be required. Most rural health care is provided in small ambulatory practice settings and small hospitals, many of which are financially fragile and have limited access to capital for investing in EHRs. Rural health systems are also more dependent than urban systems on public payment programs, such as Medicaid, safety net grant programs for community and rural health clinics, and Medicare. In rural areas, such as Indian reservations, the federal government may also be the dominant provider of services.

Recommendation 10. Congress should provide appropriate direction and financial resources to assist rural providers in converting to electronic health records over the next 5 years. Working collaboratively with the Office of the National Coordinator for Health Information Technology:

- The Indian Health Service should develop a strategy for transitioning all of its provider sites (including those operated by tribal governments under the Self-Determination Act) from paper to electronic health records.
- The Health Resources and Services Administration should develop a strategy for transitioning community health centers, rural health clinics, critical access hospitals, and other rural providers from paper to electronic health records.
- The Centers for Medicare and Medicaid Services and the state governments should consider providing financial rewards to providers participating in Medicare or Medicaid programs that invest in electronic health records. These two large public insurance programs should work together to re-examine their benefit and payment programs to ensure appropriate coverage of telehealth and other health services delivered electronically.

The ultimate goal is to establish a national and even global health information infrastructure that allows for the exchange of patient data between authorized users in a secure environment. The NHII will likely be built community by community, with local or regional health information infrastructures adhering to national data standards. In October 2004, the Agency for Healthcare Research and Quality awarded $139 million in contracts and grants to communities and health systems to enhance ICT capabilities. The committee applauds this effort, but is concerned that current funding is too limited.

Recommendation 11. The Agency for Healthcare Research and Quality's Health Information Technology Program should be expanded. Adequate resources should be provided to allow the agency to sponsor developmental programs for information and communications technology in five rural areas. Communities should be selected from across the range of rural environments, including frontier areas. The 5-year developmental programs should commence in fiscal year 2006 and result in the establishment of state-of-the-art information and communications technology infrastructure that is accessible to all providers and all consumers in those communities.

Rural communities, like urban areas, are embarking on a period of enormous change. Communities will need both technical and educational assistance to make this transition smoothly and successfully.

Recommendation 12. The National Library of Medicine, in collaboration with the Office of the National Coordinator for Health Information Technology and the Agency for Healthcare Research and Quality,
should establish regional information and communications technol-
ogy/telehealth resource centers that are interconnected with the National Network of Libraries of Medicine. These resource centers should
provide a full spectrum of services, including the following:

- Information resources for health professionals and consumers,
including access to online information sources and technical assistance with online applications, such as distance monitoring.
- Lifelong educational programs for health care professionals.
- An on-call resource center to assist communities in resolving
technical, organizational, clinical, financial, and legal questions related to information and communications technology.

SUMMARY

Rural communities should focus on improving both personal and population health programs to realize the greatest improvement in health and
health care. An integrated approach to identifying priorities and allocating
resources is needed. It will also be necessary to cultivate a new cadre of
health care leaders capable of viewing clinical care within the broader
context of population health and building communitywide collaborative
structures.

The federal government should establish a Rural Quality Initiative to
assist rural communities and providers in acquiring the knowledge and tools
needed to improve quality. Steps should be taken immediately to ensure that
rural communities are not left behind in the many quality-related initiatives,
including standardized performance measurement, public reporting, and
pay-for-performance programs.

It will also be important to remain vigilant in addressing long-standing
shortages of health professionals pursuing practice in rural settings, while at
the same time taking steps to better prepare health professionals to provide
quality care in rural environments. ICT is a transformational tool that has
great potential to improve health and health care. Federal financial and technical assistance will be required to ensure that rural providers transition
from paper to electronic health records, and that rural communities benefit
fully from the ICT infrastructure being built over the coming decade.

REFERENCES

IOM (Institute of Medicine). 1990. *Medicare: A Strategy for Quality Assurance, Volume I.* Washington, DC: National Academy Press. P. 4.

IOM. 2003. *Fostering Rapid Advances in Health Care: Learning from System Demonstrations.* Washington, DC: The National Academies Press.

1

Introduction

A sense of distinction between rural and urban settings and communities is of long standing. The playwright Euripides is said to have offered the view in the 5th century BC that "The first prerequisite to happiness is that a man be born in a famous city." And in the 3rd century BC, the writer of Ecclesiasticus, a book of the Apocrypha, asked the question "How can he get wisdom who holdeth the plow?" Yet in the formative age of our country, it was the virtues of agrarianism that were strongly asserted by Thomas Jefferson, who referred scathingly to the "mobs of great cities" and called farmers "the chosen people of God" (Beale and Cromartie, 2004, p. 1).

Rural communities are a vital, diverse component of the United States, representing nearly 20 percent of the nation's population. The basic demographic feature of a rural area is that it is a place of low population density and small aggregate size. There is no one standard definition of rural in terms of population statistics. The most long-standing U.S. definition has been that of the Census Bureau, which defines rural as open country and settlements of less than 2,500 residents, exclusive of embedded suburbs of urbanized areas of 50,000 or more population. The Office of Management and Budget and the Economic Research Service have somewhat similar definitions (see Appendix B). Frontier areas are considered the most thinly settled counties, with population densities of fewer than 7 households per square mile.

Rural America reflects the multiethnicity of the nation as a whole. African American communities are numerous across the South's lowland districts; Native Americans are clustered in the northern High Plains, the Four Corners region in the Southwest, and Alaska; and significant numbers of Hispanics live in the rural counties along the Rio Grande Valley.

There are, however, important differences between rural and urban areas that affect the delivery of health care services. Rural areas tend to have an older age structure than urban areas, as younger people migrate from rural areas and as retired people move in. This characteristic has implications for

19

the health care infrastructure: the elderly have a greater need for health care services, especially for chronic disease management and long-term care. Rural populations also exhibit poorer health behaviors (i.e., higher rates of smoking and obesity and lower rates of exercise). Compared with urban residents, rural populations tend to have lower levels of income and education and higher rates of unemployment. Further, uninsurance rates are higher in rural than in urban counties. Thus, in rural areas there is a greater need for health care safety net providers. Finally, distances to health care providers are longer in rural areas.

Rural areas have a strong sense of community responsibility and propensity toward collaboration. As a result, they are adept at devising unique and creative ways to build social and physical infrastructures needed to provide the services that urban areas take for granted.

Generally, there are fewer health care organizations and professionals of all kinds in rural areas, and the availability of health care services varies widely. Some rural communities adjacent to urban centers have access to the full range of health care services, while remote villages and isolated towns may have few if any medical resources. Those providers that are located in rural areas are characterized by less choice and competition, and some have broadened their scope of practice to accommodate the needs of the local community. For most rural communities, retaining workforce capacity and health care services—whether primary care, emergency, hospital care, long-term care, mental health and substance abuse, oral health, or public health—has been a continuing challenge.

RURAL HEALTH POLICY

Making correct decisions on rural health policy is contingent on understanding the unique characteristics of the communities and conditions in which health care is delivered. Rural communities are heterogeneous, differing in population density, remoteness from urban areas, and the cultural norms of the regions of which they are part. As a result, they vary in their demographic, environmental, economic, and social characteristics. These differences influence the magnitude and types of health problems communities face.

National health policy has been increasingly responsive to rural health needs and problems. Over the years since 1983, Congress has created special categories of rural hospitals that receive either cost-based payment or elevated Medicare payments: rural referral centers, sole community hospitals, Medicare-dependent hospitals, and, in 1997, critical access hospitals. More recently, the Medicare Prescription Drug Improvement and Modernization Act of 2003 introduced a more favorable financial climate for rural hospitals.

Partly in response to these changes, there has been a renaissance in rural health care in a number of rural communities. Some rural hospitals are replacing aging facilities (Gregg et al., 2002; Howe and Bavery, 1999; Rees, 2002). There are also examples of hospitals, physicians, and other health care providers building regional networks that are giving rural residents greater access to state-of-the art health care (Gregg and Moscovice, 2003; Minyard et al., 2003; Nebraska Office of Rural Health, 2002; Novack, 2003; Rosenthal et al., 1997; User Liaison Program, 1997). In addition, some rural health care providers and communities are embarking on significant quality improvement initiatives in response to the national quality movement (see Chapter 3). But these changes have not been enough. They are not widespread, and they are occurring too slowly. Many rural communities continue to struggle to sustain viable health care delivery systems (see Appendix C). In recent years, it has also become apparent that rural communities confront serious quality of care challenges as well.

PURPOSE AND SCOPE OF THIS STUDY

In the above context and given the increased interest in the quality of health care in rural America, the Health Resources and Services Administration (HRSA), the Agency for Healthcare Research and Quality (AHRQ), and the Substance Abuse and Mental Health Services Administration (SAMHSA) of the Department of Health and Human Services (DHHS), together with the W. K. Kellogg Foundation, requested that the Institute of Medicine (IOM) undertake an independent, unbiased assessment of the condition of health and health care in rural America, and formulate an action plan for quality-focused rural community health systems. The charge to the committee included the following specific tasks:

- Assess the quality of health care in rural areas;
- Develop a conceptual framework for a core set of services and the essential infrastructure necessary to deliver those services to rural communities;
- Recommend priority objectives, and identify the changes in policies and programs needed to accomplish those objectives, including, but not

limited to, payment policies and the necessary information and communications technology infrastructure; and

- Consider implications for federal programs and policy.

In response to this request, the IOM appointed a committee of 12 members representing a range of expertise related to the scope of the study (see Appendix A for biographical sketches of committee members). The committee addressed its charge by reviewing the salient research literature, published and unpublished; government reports and data; empirical evidence; and additional materials provided by government officials and others. In addition, a workshop was held to augment the committee's knowledge and expertise through more focused discussion of specific issues of concern, and to obtain input from a wide range of researchers, providers of health services, and interested members of the public. The committee also commissioned four background papers to avail itself of expert, detailed, and independent analysis of some of the key issues beyond the time and resources of its members (Beale and Cromartie, 2004; Gamm and Hutchison, 2004; Mueller and McBride, 2004; Nesbitt et al., 2004).

The scope of the committee's charge was very broad, covering the full range of health care services for people residing in different rural settings. The committee recognizes the growing importance of ensuring a broad range of quality health care services for rural America; however, resource and time constraints, as well as a lack of sufficient data, prevented the committee from fully addressing the issues surrounding all the services, settings, and population groups that might be considered relevant to its charge. For instance, a comprehensive consideration of the availability and quality of long-term care, coordinated care for chronic diseases and disability, and quality monitoring and reporting systems need to be addressed by separate studies.

BUILDING ON IOM'S *QUALITY CHASM* SERIES

The IOM has a long history of addressing quality of care issues. This IOM committee began its work by first reviewing the sizable body of knowledge that has accumulated through the efforts of many other IOM committees. Following is a brief summary of some of the key definitions, findings, and recommendations from other IOM reports that are of particular relevance to this committee's work.

Promulgated in 1990, the IOM's definition of quality of care has stood the test of time—addressing both population- and individual-level health care needs and encompassing clinician and patient perspectives:

Quality of care is the degree to which health services for individuals and populations increase the likelihood of desired health outcomes and are consistent with current professional knowledge (IOM, 1990; p. 4).

This definition encompasses both services that clinicians deliver to individuals (e.g., preventive, diagnostic, and treatment) and services available to defined populations (e.g., health education). Health services include a wide range of physical, dental, and mental health care—preventive, acute, and long-term care—provided in all settings.

The above definition is consistent with the view that the health care system of the twenty-first century should balance and integrate the need for personal health care with broader communitywide initiatives that target the entire population and the environment (IOM, 2003a). Many factors influence the health of individuals and populations, including not only the environment, but also social behaviors and genetic predispositions (Kindig and Stoddart, 2003).

With the release of *Crossing the Quality Chasm: A New Health System for the 21st Century* in 2001, the IOM embarked on what will likely be a decade-long journey to work with others toward reform of the health care system. The *Quality Chasm* report was a clarion call to improve the American health care delivery system as a whole along all of its quality dimensions. The report identifies six aims for quality improvement: health care should be safe, effective, patient-centered, timely, efficient, and equitable (see Table 1-1). These aims have now been endorsed by leading public- and private-sector organizations involved in health care reform. The *Quality Chasm* report stresses that a major overhaul of the health care delivery system is needed, and that changes will be needed at many levels.

In 2003, the *Quality Chasm* series began focusing on the role of communities. In response to a request from the Secretary of DHHS, the IOM produced the report *Fostering Rapid Advances in Health Care: Learning from System Demonstrations* (IOM, 2003a), laying out a bottom-up strategy for health system reform that builds on the vision set forth in the *Quality Chasm* report. This strategy is based on the use of states or "market areas" as laboratories for the design, implementation, and testing of alternative strategies, leading ultimately to the creation of a set of model twenty-first-century community health systems over the coming years.

To further galvanize efforts directed at rapid-cycle experimentation at the community level, the IOM held the *1st Annual Crossing the Quality Chasm Summit: A Focus on Communities* in January 2004 (IOM, 2004). Fifteen communities and many national leaders participated in this summit, which focused on the development of action plans to produce significant

TABLE 1-1 Six Aims for Quality Improvement

Aim	Definition
Safety	Avoiding injuries to patients from the care that is intended to help them
Effectiveness	Providing services based on scientific knowledge (evidence-based) to all who could benefit and refraining from providing services to those not likely to benefit (avoiding underuse and overuse, respectively)
Patient-centeredness	Providing care that is respectful of and responsive to individual patient preferences, needs, and values and ensuring that patient values guide all clinical decisions
Timeliness	Avoiding waits and sometimes harmful delays for both those who receive and those who give care
Efficiency	Avoiding waste, including waste of equipment, supplies, ideas, and energy
Equity	Providing care that does not vary in quality because of personal characteristics such as gender, ethnicity, geographic location, and socioeconomic status

SOURCE: IOM, 2001.

improvements in five of the areas identified in the IOM report *Priority Areas for National Action: Transforming Health Care Quality* (IOM, 2003b): diabetes, asthma, heart disease, depression, and pain control in advanced cancer.

The *Fostering Rapid Advances* report and the *1st Annual Crossing the Quality Chasm Summit* report reflect a growing conviction on the part of many in the health care community that the health care system is too complex and geographically diverse to be reformed through national policy alone. This committee believes that rural communities afford a unique opportunity to experiment with various rapid-innovation strategies. At the same time, implementation of these health system reforms in rural "market areas" needs to reflect the important distinctions that exist between the rural health care delivery system and its urban and suburban counterparts. As discussed below, the situation in rural communities is different from that in urban and suburban areas; thus application of the quality reform agenda to rural areas will require a different assessment of services, resources, and connectivity.

GUIDING PRINCIPLES FOR REFORMING
RURAL HEALTH CARE

In carrying out its work, the Committee on the Future of Rural Health Care confronted two challenges. The first was to determine how best to apply within a rural context the sizable body of work that has accumulated through the efforts of the IOM, as well as those of the many other public- and private-sector organizations engaged in the reform effort. The second was to contribute to the body of intellectual thought regarding health system reform in ways that will benefit all communities, both rural and urban.

The committee was guided in its deliberations by the overriding principle that *all rural Americans should have access to the full spectrum of high-quality, appropriate health care,* regardless of where they live. Within the context of rural health, the committee interpreted the above overriding principle as follows:

• *Rural communities should focus greater attention on improving population health in addition to meeting personal health care needs.* Health care is only one of a number of determinants of the health of individuals, families, and communities. Traditional and expanded public health capacity focused on such issues as the environment, school-based health, and social support for the disadvantaged and handicapped can have a major impact on community health. A major theme of this report is that health care providers share with other groups (for example, consumers, employers, educators, government, and religious organizations) the responsibility to work together to achieve population health outcomes. Collaborative efforts are needed at the community level to create environments that minimize the likelihood of illness or disease (for example, through immunization campaigns), and to provide incentives for residents to pursue healthy lifestyles (for example, encouraging regular exercise). To have the greatest impact, the health care system must have well-defined processes for targeting limited resources in pursuit of both community-level and personal health care interventions.

• *A core set of health care services (primary care, dental care, basic mental health care, and emergency medical services) should be available within rural communities.* Health care has technical, cultural, social, and emotional dimensions. Patients are best served when they receive quality health care in their home environment from providers who are sensitive to local cultural norms and values, and know patients as members of families and communities. Requiring patients to travel long distances—the costs of which generally are not reimbursed by health insurance—to receive their health care not only raises the cost and complexity of care, but also may impair outcomes by increasing the patient's physical and emotional stress, reducing the likelihood of seeking follow-up care, and limiting proximate family support. Yet not all services can be delivered locally. Rural communities may not generate a large enough volume of services for certain specialty providers to support their practices financially and to maintain adequate levels of skill and technological support to deliver safe and effective care.

• *When care cannot be delivered locally, links should be established to services in other locales.* Rural communities should have established relationships with health care providers and institutions in urban settings to provide their residents with seamless access to a full range of well-coordinated services.

• *The spectrum of services available in rural communities should be based on the population health needs of the local community.* Rural areas are heterogeneous in size, density, the demographic and socioeconomic composition of the population, and the cultural norms and values of families and the community. Whether services are provided locally or at a distance depends on a host of factors associated with the specific rural community. Each community should have a mechanism for determining the appropriate spectrum of services to maintain locally for its population, guided by the imperative that any service provided locally must be of high quality and economically feasible.

• *The provision of rural health care services should be shaped and guided by local community and rural organizations and institutions.* Although not all health care services can be provided in rural areas, rural communities can be instrumental in helping shape the health care systems on which they depend. Solutions to rural health care issues should be shaped by the structured input of rural residents. Both locally operated health systems and those that are part of networks spanning urban and rural communities should incorporate rural perspectives and local residents in their governing structures. Health literacy must be fostered in ways that acknowledge the culture of the rural population.

• *Rural health care requires a team of well-trained health care clinicians, managers, and leaders working together.* These teams must provide continuous services, maintain adequate coverage, and establish and foster seamless linkages with other elements of the health care system both locally and at a distance—a major challenge for rural health care systems. Health professions educational institutions, particularly those in states with large proportions of rural populations, have the responsibility to select, train, and support health professionals for rural practice. Health professions schools, including those for dentists and mental health professionals, have a public trust. They are supported by public funds and have an obligation to incorporate the needs of the public into their clinical and educational mission. Furthermore, they must realize that their responsibility does not end when students graduate; rather, they must work to support rural-based providers by extending continuing education opportunities and providing links to the academic environment.

- *Health care financing should explicitly address the special circumstances of rural areas.* One of the major problems facing the American health care system is the number of people who are uninsured, a problem that is complicated in rural areas by the small numbers of large employers, who traditionally offer most of the health insurance in the United States. To create the future rural health care system, mechanisms must be designed for making health insurance available for all residents, whether rural or urban. Mechanisms must also be designed for providing capital and financial support for rural health care institutions, such as hospitals and nursing homes; for rural infrastructures, such as emergency medical services and health care applications of information and communications technology; and for community-based initiatives. Major sources of public financing, such as Medicare and Medicaid, must consider the special needs of rural beneficiaries in the design and application of new policies and procedures. For example, the introduction of pay-for-performance programs must reflect the special circumstances of rural health care—the smaller scale and differing case mix as compared with urban health care.

- *Efforts to develop local and national health information technology infrastructures should focus specific attention on rural communities.* All communities stand to derive sizable benefits from the National Health Information Infrastructure, but these benefits may be even more substantial in rural communities. The development of an information and communications technology infrastructure offers much potential to provide rural residents and their local providers with virtual access to specialists in outside areas, and to enhance the access of all providers to complete patient data and information in a timely fashion. Given their limited financial resources and the small scale of rural provider organizations, most rural health care systems will need financial and technical assistance to establish electronic health records and secure platforms for data exchange.

ORGANIZATION OF THE REPORT

This report addresses the current status of health care quality in rural America and proposes ways to build quality, focused rural community health systems. Chapter 2 presents an integrated approach to addressing both population health and personal health care needs. Chapter 3 addresses quality measurement and improvement initiatives in rural areas. Chapter 4 identifies strategies for strengthening the human resources available to rural communities to improve health and health care, focusing on the availability and preparedness of health care professionals, as well as broad-based mobilization of a community's residents and key stakeholders. Chapter 5 addresses the implementation of pay-for-performance initiatives within the rural context; it also examines the financial viability of rural health care delivery systems and recent steps taken to improve rural health care financing. Finally, Chapter 6 considers ways to foster the deployment of the National Health Information Infrastructure required for the delivery of quality care, homeland security, and public health applications.

The committee hopes that this report will contribute to the development of policies leading to high-quality, efficient, and cost-effective health care systems for rural America. The report is intended to provide guidance to a wide audience, including those in rural communities working to improve health and health care, individuals responsible for national and state health policy, and those in the research community working on rural health issues.

Finally, the committee believes that broader health reform efforts focusing on both urban and rural communities would benefit from implementation of the health reform strategies proposed in this report for rural communities. Rural communities represent excellent sites to pilot innovative ways of improving population health and personal health care delivery, given the smaller scale of rural health care and the strong sense of community in rural areas. Although these pilot projects would be tailored to the rural context, many of the lessons learned would have broad applicability to other communities.

REFERENCES

Beale C, Cromartie J. 2004 (February). *Profile of the Rural Population.* Commissioned Paper for the IOM Committee on the Future of Rural Health Care. Washington, DC.

Gamm L, Hutchison L. 2004 (February). *Mental Health and Substance Abuse Services: Prospects for Rural Communities.* Commissioned Paper for the IOM Committee on the Future of Rural Health Care. Washington, DC.

Gregg W, Moscovice I. 2003. The evolution of rural health networks: Implications for health care managers. *Health Care Management Review* 28(2):161–177.

Gregg W, Knott A, Moscovice I. 2002. *Rural Hospital Access to Capital: Issues and Recommendations.* Minneapolis, MN: Rural Health Research Center, University of Minnesota.

Howe P, Bavery G. 1999. Funding for renovation: A rural hospital's experience. *Seminars in Perioperative Nursing* 8(4):229–232.

IOM (Institute of Medicine). 1990. *Medicare: A Strategy for Quality Assurance, Volume I.* Washington, DC: National Academy Press. P. 4.

IOM. 2001. *Crossing the Quality Chasm: A New Health System for the 21st Century.* Washington, DC: National Academy Press.

IOM. 2003a. *Fostering Rapid Advances in Health Care: Learning from System Demonstrations.* Washington, DC: The National Academies Press.

IOM. 2003b. *Priority Areas for National Action: Transforming Health Care Quality.* Washington, DC: The National Academies Press.

IOM. 2004. *1st Annual Crossing the Quality Chasm Summit: A Focus on Communities.* Washington, DC: The National Academies Press.

Kindig D, Stoddart GL. 2003. What is population health? *American Journal of Public Health* 93(3):380–383.

Minyard KJ, Lineberry IC, Smith TA, Byrd-Roubides T. 2003. Transforming the delivery of rural health care in Georgia: State partnership strategy for developing rural health networks. *Journal of Rural Health* 19(Supplement):361–371.

Mueller KJ, McBride, TD. 2004 (February). *Financing the Rural Health Care Delivery System.* Commissioned Paper for the IOM Committee on the Future of Rural Health Care. Washington, DC.

Nebraska Office of Rural Health. 2002. *Nebraska's Story: A Collection of Nine Critical Access Hospital Community Stories and Two Network Stories.* Lincoln, NE: Nebraska Department of Health and Human Services, Office of Rural Health.

Nesbitt TS, Yellowlees PM, Hogarth M, Hilty DM. 2004 (March). *Rural Health Care in the Digital Age: The Role of Information and Telecommunications Technologies in the Future of Rural Health.* Commissioned Paper for the IOM Committee on the Future of Rural Health Care. Washington, DC.

Novack, NL. 2003 (September). *Bridging the Gap in Rural Healthcare. The Main Street Economist: Commentary on the Rural Economy.* [Online]. Available: http://www.kc.frb.org/RuralCenter/mainstreet/MSE_0903.pdf [accessed July 2004].

Rees T. 2002. North Carolina hospital redefines itself as a critical-access facility. Bertie Memorial called a national model. *Profiles in Healthcare Marketing* 18(1):34–39.

Rosenthal TC, James P, Fox C, Wysong J, FitzPatrick PG. 1997. Rural physicians, rural networks, and free market health care in the 1990s. *Archives of Family Medicine* 6(4):319–323.

User Liaison Program. 1997 (November 19–21). *Strengthening the Rural Health Infrastructure: Network Development and Managed Care Strategies—Workshop Summary.* [Online]. Available: http://www.ahrq.gov/new/ulp/ulpstren.htm [accessed August 2004].

2

An Integrated Approach to Improving Health and Health Care in Rural Communities

SUMMARY

This chapter provides an integrated approach to addressing the personal health care and population health needs of rural communities. The six quality aims of the Institute of Medicine's Crossing the Quality Chasm: A New Health System for the 21st Century *are used to illustrate the broad range of actions that might be taken by rural communities at both the level of the personal health care system and the community level to improve health status. Many community-level actions extend beyond the traditional health care sector, thus necessitating greater collaboration between that sector and others, such as education, transportation, and social services. By making explicit the full range of options available to rural communities for improving health, the integrated framework set forth in this chapter is intended to lead closer to a more optimal allocation of scarce financial resources between personal health care and population health initiatives.*

In 2001, the Institute of Medicine (IOM) released the report, *Crossing the Quality Chasm: A New Health System for the 21st Century,* calling for fundamental reform of the nation's health care system. As the report makes clear, an extensive body of evidence substantiates the existence of a large quality gap—the care people actually receive falls far short of the care they should receive.

This IOM committee concurs with earlier IOM committees that fundamental change in the health care delivery system is needed to improve the quality of care and ultimately the health status of the population. But this will not be enough. Although access to high-quality personal health care services (e.g., preventive, acute, chronic, and end-of-life care) increases health and reduces pain and suffering, there are other determinants of health status in a community. Health outcomes are determined to a great extent by genetic predispositions, health behaviors, environmental exposures or threats, and social circumstances (e.g., educational levels, socioeconomic status) (LaLonde, 1975; McGinnis et al., 2002).

Moreover, a growing body of research demonstrates the importance of considering these factors within a community context (Hillemeier et al., 2003). There is much variability across communities in terms of population health needs. Communities also have different strengths and resources to bring to bear in addressing population health needs. Lastly, addressing population health needs often requires strong local leadership and collaboration across different sectors and multiple stakeholders within a community.

This chapter presents an integrated approach to addressing both personal health care and population health needs that builds on the six quality aims of the *Quality Chasm* report. The approach is intended to be most useful at the community level in facilitating prioritization of a community's health needs and identification of the most promising interventions. The first section reviews the rather limited amount of literature that is available on the quality of rural health care. The second section addresses population health priorities in rural areas, with emphasis on the unique aspects of rural communities that should be considered in shaping a reform strategy. The third section proposes an integrated framework for addressing both personal health care and population health needs in rural communities, providing examples of interventions at both the community and individual levels that might contribute to improved population health. The fourth and final section summarizes the IOM committee's conclusions and recommendations for moving forward.

QUALITY OF CARE IN RURAL COMMUNITIES

As noted above, there is a large body of evidence documenting serious shortcomings in the American health care system for each of the six quality aims identified in the *Quality Chasm* report. In 2000, the IOM published the report *To Err Is Human: Building a Safer Health System,* calling national attention to the tens of thousands of Americans who die each year as a result of medical errors. A year later, the IOM released the *Quality Chasm* report, calling for fundamental reform of the nation's health care system. Both reports include literature reviews. An appendix to the *Quality Chasm* report provides a literature review conducted by researchers at the RAND Corporation based on 73 publications from peer-reviewed journals. These literature reviews substantiate the existence of a large quality gap: the care people actually receive falls far short of the care they should receive.

Since the release of these reports, numerous other publications have documented the serious nature of the quality challenge. Studies continue to reveal disturbing rates of medical errors in virtually all health care settings—hospital, nursing home, and ambulatory (Gurwitz et al., 2000, 2003). In addition to studies focusing on safety, recent evidence raises concerns about the effectiveness of health care. Of particular note, a large research study conducted by RAND found that, on average, patients receive only about 55 percent of those services from which they would likely benefit (McGlynn et al., 2003).

Much of this research on quality of care has been conducted in urban settings. Some of the large analyses have included rural providers in their study samples, but have not reported rural-specific results (see, for example, Thomas et al., 1999). There is no reason to believe that the *overall* results (i.e., that quality is highly variable) of this large body of literature would not apply to rural America, as the factors believed to contribute to these quality shortcomings (e.g., poorly designed systems, siloed delivery systems, inadequate use of information technology) exist to varying degrees in both rural and urban areas. But there may well be rural and urban differences in the prevalence of particular types of quality problems, not to mention the specific approaches that would be most effective in improving quality.

As the overall literature on the state of quality has been examined in previous IOM reports, it is not reviewed in this report. However, a small number of studies exist comparing quality in rural and urban areas, and these are reviewed in this section. Also discussed are studies that point to the need for different types of interventions in rural versus urban settings to address concerns regarding quality of health care. The discussion is organized according to the six quality aims set forth in Chapter 2 of the *Quality Chasm* report.

Safety

Patient safety is the prevention of harm to patients (IOM, 2004). In a recent comparison of rural and urban hospitals using 19 safety measures,

Romano and colleagues found that rural hospitals had lower risk-adjusted rates of potential safety-related events for 14 of the 19 indicators (e.g., decubitus ulcer, infection due to medical care, postoperative respiratory failure), and higher rates for 5 indicators (anesthesia reactions and complications, accidental puncture and laceration, postoperative hip fracture, abdominopelvic wound dehiscence, and birth trauma) (Jolliffe, 2003; Romano et al., 2003). An earlier study of New York state hospitals found that rural hospitals had significantly lower adverse event rates than New York City and urban upstate hospitals after controlling for age and severity of illness (Whitener and McGranahan, 2003). Another study examined rural hospitals by bed size and found that, compared with large rural hospitals (100+ beds), both medium-sized (50–99 beds) and small (<50 beds) rural hospitals had significantly lower rates of postoperative hip fracture, hemorrhage, and hematoma; the medium-sized hospitals had lower rates of postoperative respiratory failure, while the small hospitals had lower rates of iatrogenic pneumothorax infection (Cromartie, 2002). On the other hand, a study of rural health clinics documented a wide range of medication errors, including errors in dosage, errors in agent selection, and failure to recognize potential drug interactions and contraindications (Williamson et al., 1991).

Patient safety practices are processes or structures whose application reduces the probability of adverse events resulting from exposure to the health care system across a range of diseases and procedures (Shojania et al., 2002). Since the publication of the IOM reports *To Err Is Human* (IOM, 2000) and *Crossing the Quality Chasm* (IOM, 2001), key organizations involved in patient safety activities have augmented their programs. For example, the National Quality Forum (NQF) has endorsed standards to improve patient safety, the Agency for Healthcare Research and Quality (AHRQ) has published evidence-based studies on specific actions that can increase patient safety, and the Joint Commission on Accreditation of Healthcare Organizations (JCAHO) has expanded initiatives and resources to enhance patient safety in the organizations it accredits (NQF, 2003; AHRQ, 2004; JCAHO, 2004). In addition, health care purchasers, notably represented by the Leapfrog Group, have developed several targeted standards for delivering care to increase safety.

Nonetheless, there is a general absence of studies examining patient safety issues in rural provider settings. Of the few research studies that do exist (Coburn et al., forthcoming; Romano et al., 2003), there has been no evaluation of how the characteristics of rural practice, such as smaller-sized facilities and low volume, may impact patient safety. In addition, rural providers may face different safety risks. For example, given the more limited services available in rural areas, patients are more likely to be referred or transferred for diagnosis and treatment. The interfaces between personnel at different facilities, the application of standardized protocols, and the transfer of complete and relevant information all require significant attention to minimize the potential for error and ensure seamless transfers.

Effectiveness

Effectiveness refers to care that is evidence-based (IOM, 2001). Evidence-based practice is the integration of the best research evidence with clinical expertise and patient values (Sackett et al., 1996). Such care avoids both overuse, or the provision of services that expose the patient to more potential harm than good, and underuse, or the failure to provide services from which the patient would likely have benefited (Wisconsin Medical Society, 2002).

The evidence pertaining to rural and urban differences in effectiveness is mixed. One study found that rural areas scored higher than urban on the appropriate provision of preventive services related to breast examinations/ family history for breast cancer, influenza immunization, and cholesterol screening; no differences were found in provision of preventive services for blood pressure, tobacco use screening and counseling, and mammography and pap smears (Pol et al., 2001). On the other hand, rural populations tend to be diagnosed at a more advanced stage of cancer, to be less likely to have their cancer staged at the time of diagnosis, and to have less access to state-of-the-art technology (Gamm et al., 2002). A study of elderly diabetic patients found that patients in large remote rural communities (i.e., ones that could support both generalist and specialist physicians) were significantly more likely to receive those services than their urban counterparts, while patients in smaller rural communities were less likely to receive those services than urban patients (Rosenblatt et al., 2001).

One study of interventions for acute myocardial infarction (AMI) found that patients admitted to rural hospitals were less likely to receive aspirin, heparin, intravenous (IV) nitroglycerin, and IV fluids (Baldwin et al., 2004). In another study, Medicare beneficiaries hospitalized for AMI in rural hospitals were found to be less likely than those hospitalized in urban hospitals to receive several recommended interventions (e.g., aspirin, heparin, IV nitroglycerin), and risk-adjusted rates of death within 30 days of an admission for an AMI increased with "rurality" or degree of remoteness of the hospital

(Baldwin et al., 2004). An analysis of outcomes of coronary angioplasty procedures performed in rural and urban hospitals found that in-hospital mortality after angioplasty for AMI was worse in low- and medium-volume rural hospitals, but overall outcomes in rural and urban hospitals were similar for patients without infarction (Maynard et al., 2000).

Patient-Centeredness

Care that is patient-centered reflects the qualities of compassion, empathy, and responsiveness to the needs, values, and expressed preferences of the individual patient (IOM, 2001). Patient-centeredness is a multifaceted concept that incorporates such elements as the following:

- Patient satisfaction with care
- Provision of information, education, and other supports to assist patients in self-management of chronic conditions (Lorig et al., 1999; Wagner, 1998)
- Efforts to promote patient health literacy (Detmer et al., 2003)
- Shared decision making between patients and clinicians

Few studies have assessed differences in patient perceptions of these qualities in rural and urban areas. One study did find that rural providers generally score higher on compassion and accessibility than their urban counterparts, but many believe that rural physicians are less qualified (Reiber et al., 1996).

Timeliness

Timeliness in access to care is a critical factor influencing the quality of rural health care. While timeliness in the urban sense tends to denote long waits at doctors' offices or emergency rooms or waiting on gurneys in hallways for procedures, in the rural context, timeliness often reflects the response times of emergency medical personnel and the overall distance a patient must travel to receive services.

Timely access to emergency care is a major issue for rural residents. Response times by emergency medical personnel and transport times via ambulance to the hospital are notably greater than in urban areas. A study of five counties in Washington State found the mean response time for rural incidents was 13.6 minutes (median = 12 minutes), versus 7 minutes (median = 6 minutes) for urban incidents (Grossman et al., 1997). Mean transport times were also significantly longer for rural incidents (17.2 minutes in rural areas versus 8.2 minutes for urban), and death risk was seven times higher if the response time was greater than 30 minutes. Another study of 12 counties near Augusta, Georgia, found more modest differences with rural and urban emergency response times of 7.9 and 5.1 minutes, respectively (Morrisey et al., 1995). Handoffs between clinicians at each point along the response continuum have a significant impact on the outcome of rural patients because of the overall fragmentation of emergency medical services and the rural health system in general, and the greater geographic distances that must be traveled to reach the local emergency room or nearby trauma center.

Timeliness also relates to the long distances patients must travel to receive health care services because of the scarcity of human and technological resources in the local community. When local resources are inadequate to provide core health care services to the population, the quality of health care suffers. One study of 16 rural areas with high outflow of patients to urban centers found that poor local access to providers of obstetric care was associated with a significantly greater risk of having an abnormal neonate for both Medicaid and privately insured rural patients (Nesbitt et al., 2004). Another study of rural adults with HIV infection found that nearly 75 percent sought care in urban areas and that more than 25 percent had delayed obtaining care in the past 6 months because of travel considerations (Ormond et al., 2000).

Efficiency

Efficient health systems optimize resources and minimize waste to obtain the best value for investments in health care services and administration. Efficient systems ensure that the appropriate clinical services are available to meet the health needs of the local community while balancing cost of care and avoiding underuse, overuse, and misuse of services (IOM, 2001).

Comparisons of efficiency between rural and urban health systems can be misleading. Efficiency is a measure of inputs over desired outputs, and if one of the outputs is care close to home, comparisons of efficiency need to have a rural-to-rural rather than rural-to-urban focus. The committee realizes it is not feasible to provide all health care services close to home, but this should be the goal for the core services (i.e., primary care in the community, emergency medical services, primary- and secondary-level hospital care, long-term care, mental health and substance abuse services, oral health care, and public health services).

It is also important to recognize that rural and urban health care delivery systems have different advantages and disadvantages when delivering care. Rural systems are generally less complex than urban, so certain types of inefficiencies, such as the ordering of redundant laboratory tests because the results of earlier tests cannot be located, may occur less frequently. Conversely, larger urban providers likely benefit from volume discounts when purchasing supplies, material, and other resources.

Equity

The aim of equity is to ensure that the availability of care and quality of services are based on an individual's health care needs and not on personal characteristics such as gender, ethnicity, geographic location, and socioeconomic status (IOM, 2001). Differences in the availability of health care resources (see Chapter 4) between rural and urban areas are one form of inequity noted throughout this report. Rural areas, like urban, also confront equity issues related to the sizable numbers of residents who do not have health insurance or have insurance that provides very limited coverage. There is a sizable body of evidence indicating that people who lack health insurance receive too little health care, and often the services they do receive are not timely (IOM, 2002). These studies are not specific to rural areas, however, so it is not possible to determine whether rural areas differ from urban in terms of this equity challenge. The federal government did recently establish the Community Access Program to provide grants to rural and urban communities to expand and coordinate safety net services for uninsured and underinsured Americans (HRSA, 2004). It is too early to assess the impact of this program, but grant awards in fiscal years 2000 to 2002 totaled about $255 million. In 2002, this program was replaced by the new Healthy Communities Access Program, to which Congress appropriated $105 million for fiscal year 2003.

The IOM report *Unequal Treatment: Confronting Racial and Ethnic Disparities in Health Care* (IOM, 2003a) documents the pervasive nature of another form of inequity: disparities in the care that is received within a health system depending upon an individual's race or ethnicity. On the whole, racial and ethnic minorities tend to receive a lower quality of health care than nonminorities across a range of illnesses and health care services, even when socioeconomic factors are controlled. As discussed in Appendix

B, some minorities, such as Native Americans, Hispanics, and African Americans, are more concentrated in rural and frontier areas and have lower health status than other residents of these communities. Information is not available to indicate whether these within-system inequities are greater or lesser in rural than in urban health systems.

Summary

The evidence base pertaining to differences in quality between rural and urban health care is highly inadequate, and more research on this issue is clearly needed. In the case of safety and effectiveness, there are so few studies that it is not possible to determine whether there are differences between rural and urban areas. Timeliness is the only aim for which the results are clear and not surprising: access to critical services, such as emergency care, is impeded by geography and scarcity of providers. As for the other aims—patient-centeredness, efficiency, and equity—the evidence is anecdotal at best.

HEALTH BEHAVIORS AND HEALTH THREATS IN RURAL COMMUNITIES

A comprehensive review of the *Quality Chasm* six aims is beyond the scope of this report; however, this section highlights some of the more salient differences between rural and urban communities in terms of health behaviors and environmental threats—the two areas most amenable to intervention in the short run. Appendix B speaks to differences in the racial and ethnic compositions of rural and urban communities (which influence genetic predispositions to a great extent) and many other socioeconomic factors that influence health.

Although the evidence base pertaining to the quality of health care is lean, there is a good deal of evidence pointing to differences in the health behaviors of rural and urban populations. A recently published document, *Health, United States, 2001 with Urban and Rural Chartbook* (NCHS, 2001) highlights some of the key differences:

• Adolescents and adults living in rural counties are more likely to smoke than those in urban areas. In the most remote rural areas, about 19 percent of adolescents smoke, as compared with 11 percent of adolescents in metropolitan central areas. Adults living in the most rural counties are the most likely to smoke (27 percent of women and 31 percent of men), and those living in large metropolitan areas are the least likely (20 percent of women and 24–25 percent of men).

• Remote rural areas have the highest rates of self-reported obesity among women of all geographic areas. About 23 percent of female residents in rural counties are obese as compared with 16 percent of those living in metropolitan fringe areas (i.e., suburban) and 20 percent of those in metropolitan central areas.

• Residents of very rural areas (no city with a population of 10,000 or greater) are the most likely to be inactive during leisure time, followed by central city residents of large metropolitan areas. Lack of regular physical exercise is particularly high in nonmetropolitan counties of the South, where 56 percent of women and 53 percent of men report that they do not engage in exercise, sports, or physically active hobbies during leisure time. These rates are very high compared with national rates for metropolitan fringe areas (28 percent for men and 34 percent for women).

There are also differences in the threats to health that are present in rural and urban communities. For example, deaths from unintentional injuries (e.g., motor vehicle injuries, falls, poisoning, and suffocation) increase as counties become less urban (NCHS, 2001). In 1996–1998, the age-adjusted death rate for unintentional injury for males was 86 percent higher in most rural counties than in the fringe counties of large metropolitan areas. For females, this rate was about 80 percent higher in the most rural counties than in large metropolitan (central and fringe) counties.

In summary, important health behaviors and health threats can and should be addressed at the community level to achieve an optimal impact on health status. There are sizable differences between rural and urban areas in both of these regards, and these differences need to be better understood. Moreover, important differences are likely to exist within rural communities in terms of priorities for action, necessitating community- or state-based action plans.

IMPROVING POPULATION HEALTH AND PERSONAL HEALTH CARE

Rural America has struggled for many decades with shortages of health professionals; constrained access to specialty services; and financial, geographic, and other barriers to health care access (see Appendix C). Although addressing the problems of the availability of and access to health care services has been the cornerstone of rural health policy, an underresourced health care delivery infrastructure persists in many rural areas. The committee believes more must be done to strengthen the rural health care delivery infrastructure to achieve and sustain high-quality care, and subsequent chapters of this report provide guidance on enhancing quality improvement processes (Chapter 3), enhancing the health professions workforce (Chapter 4), providing more stable financing (Chapter 5), and building a stronger information and communications technology (ICT) infrastructure (Chapter 6). Achieving consistent, high-quality care is predicated on addressing each of these key areas.

Bolstering the personal health care delivery system is important, but the committee also believes a better balance must be struck between investments in personal health care and community health improvement strategies. As pointed out in the IOM report *Fostering Rapid Advances in Health Care: Learning from System Demonstrations:*

> The health care system of the 21st century should maximize the health and functioning of both individual patients and communities. To accomplish this goal, the system should balance and integrate needs for personal health care with broader communitywide initiatives that target the entire population. The health care system must have well-defined processes for making the best use of limited resources (IOM, 2003b, p. 19).

The committee believes rural communities must build a population health focus into decision making within the health care sector, as well as in other key areas (e.g., religious institutions, agricultural extensions, rural cooperatives, education, community and environmental planning) that influence population health. Most important, rural communities must reorient their quality improvement strategies from an exclusively patient- and provider-centric approach to one that also addresses the problems and needs of rural communities and populations.

The committee encourages rural health communities to focus greater attention and resources on improving population health. Programs focused on population health often involve collaboration, which may include providers within the health care sector. For example, the providers in a community might pool resources to sponsor a communitywide educational program aimed at the prevention and early diagnosis and treatment of diabetes. In other instances, the collaboration might involve health care providers and stakeholders outside the traditional health care sector in efforts to improve population health. For example, initiatives to reduce obesity in children might include outreach to school leadership to encourage the removal of soft drink machines and the provision of more nutritious lunches and snacks. In many rural communities, agricultural extensions and rural cooperatives represent an important resource for communicating about and educating the community's residents in key health issues.

In both cases, the leadership for such efforts must come from the health care sector (see Chapter 4). It is necessary to cultivate a new cadre of health care leaders who will be capable of viewing clinical care within the broader context of population health (Kazandjian, 2003). To support health care leaders in their efforts to focus both the health care sector and the community at large on improving population health, quality measurement and improvement systems must address the full continuum of performance measures, from health care processes to population health status.

To guide its work, the committee developed a framework designed to facilitate a more integrated approach to decision making regarding personal and community health programs and needs. As noted earlier, the *Quality Chasm* report focuses largely on health care quality within the personal health care delivery system. Using the six quality aims set forth in that report as a fundamental organizing framework, the committee first developed definitions for the aims that address population health. The committee then identified a set of illustrative performance measures and associated strategies for quality improvement at the community level to improve population health. The following discussion illustrates the use of this framework in informing key choices that must be made among rural health care quality improvement strategies. Tables 2-1 through 2-6 list the definitions, performance measures, and strategies for each of the six aims.

Safety

At the population level, safety refers to the avoidance of accidents and injuries due to hazards in the community (see Table 2-1). Environmental, occupational, recreational, and other accidents and injuries represent significant problems in rural areas, with large health and health care cost consequences. Currently, investments in programs to address these problems pale in comparison with expenditures for hospital and other health services to treat the consequences of these accidents and injuries. The question is whether this balance of expenditures is appropriate, or more resources should be directed at interventions to improve safety in the workplace and in the community overall.

TABLE 2-1 Personal Health Care System and Community-Level Interventions: Illustrative Examples for Safety

Definition		Measures		Interventions	
Personal Health Focus	Population Health Focus	Personal Health Care System	Community Level	Personal Health Care System	Community Level
Avoid injuries to patients from health care	Avoid accidents and injuries from hazards in the community	Rates of adverse drug events in hospitals due to errors in prescribing, dosing, and administering medications	Agricultural and motor vehicle injury rates Mining, quarrying, forestry, drilling, animal husbandry, agricultural, and construction occupational injury rates	Implementation of computerized medication order entry systems	Public education to encourage safe practices (e.g., seatbelt use, speed control), community planning to enhance traffic safety, and enforcement of traffic laws Worker education programs to encourage safe practices and enforcement of occupational health and safety laws

Illustrative measures of the safety of the personal health care system include inpatient and outpatient medication-related adverse drug events and nosocomial infection rates. At the population level, safety measures might include accident rates for the major occupational sectors in rural areas (e.g., mining, quarrying, forestry, agriculture, animal husbandry, oil and gas drilling, and construction) and measures of toxic environmental exposure/risk (e.g., chemical exposures). Patient-level safety improvement strategies include interventions to address medication, diagnostic, and other errors in inpatient and outpatient health care settings. A variety of community planning strategies exists for improving community-level safety, ranging from remediation of environmental hazards to enhancement of traffic safety.

Effectiveness

Rural health systems of the twenty-first century must be designed to promote not only evidence-based patient care services, but also community health improvement interventions that have been demonstrated to improve quality and health outcomes. The challenge is to improve the quality and safety of the care received by individuals through the medical care system while at the same time expanding investments in community health programs.

Although these are not zero-sum choices, the committee believes there will be increasing pressure on health care providers, policy makers, and others to demonstrate the cost-effectiveness of current patterns of health care use and quality and new investments in health care facilities, technologies, and services. Although the nation's per capita health spending far exceeds that of any other industrialized country, the United States does not consistently outperform other countries in terms of many measures of population health status and health care quality (Anderson and Hussey, 2001; Hussey et al., 2004; Reinhardt et al., 2004; WHO, 2000).

Yet setting priorities among potential population- and personal-level interventions to improve health will not be easy. To guide such decisions, it will be necessary to have data with which to assess the quality, outcomes, and cost of potential interventions at both the individual and community levels. Table 2-2 lists some measures that span these two dimensions and can guide decision making on health system reform to achieve improved quality and outcomes.

TABLE 2-2 Personal Health Care System and Community-Level Interventions: Illustrative Examples for Effectiveness

	Definition		Measures		Interventions	
	Personal Health Focus	Population Health Focus	Personal Health Care System	Community Level	Personal Health Care System	Community Level
	Provide health care services and interventions based on scientific knowledge	Pursue communitywide interventions to enhance health that are based on scientific knowledge	Percent of diabetic patients who had an annual eye and foot exam and percent of patients with normal blood glucose levels	Incidence and prevalence of obesity and diabetes in the residents of a rural community	Enhanced follow-up for obese and/or diabetic patients to improve compliance with practice guidelines and treatment regimens	Use of evidence-based community-level strategies to decrease obesity, such as community planning to encourage exercise and public policies that encourage schools to provide nutritious food

Patient- or Community-Centeredness

This important aim has both an individual and a community context. At the individual level, patient-centered care is defined by the responsiveness of health care providers and the personal health care system to individual needs, values, and preferences. In the community context, this aim reflects the degree to which all public and private stakeholders, such as education, business, transportation, and health care, are responsive to the aggregate needs, values, and preferences of the community. In the current health system and health policy framework, explicit choices are rarely made between individual and community (or societal) preferences, needs, and values. Health reform must target interventions and strategies that reflect a balanced approach to achieve both patient- and community-centeredness.

Measures of the patient-centeredness of the personal health care system include patient satisfaction with services received and interactions with providers. Measures of community-centeredness might include the extent to which health care programs and services are available to meet community health care needs, the availability of parks and recreational facilities, and public policies regarding smoking.

Another measure that might be used to assess progress in achieving this aim at the community level is the extent to which community priorities have been identified and considered in community health improvement planning and investment decisions. This measure is especially important as it reflects the concept of involving citizens in assessing how they believe the interests of individuals and communities should be balanced, particularly, but not exclusively, with regard to health services.

The strategies for quality improvement listed in Table 2-3 are only illustrative of the many that might be employed. To achieve the goal of a health system that recognizes and responds to community preferences, needs, and values, new systems of state and regional health planning will be needed that can provide a political and economic context for involving citizens and communities in critical decisions concerning health reform and quality improvement. Health professions training programs are also critical to the production of clinicians who understand and can apply the skills needed to address this goal.

Timeliness

At the level of the personal health care delivery system, timeliness refers to the reduction of waits and harmful delays in accessing health care and in

TABLE 2-3 Personal Health Care System and Community-Level Interventions: Illustrative Examples for Patient- and Community-Centeredness

Definition		Measures		Interventions	
Personal Health Focus	Population Health Focus	Personal Health Care System	Community Level	Personal Health Care System	Community Level
Provide care that is respectful of and responsive to patient preferences, needs, and values	Ensure that public- and private-sector stakeholders (e.g., education, business, transportation, health care) are respectful of and responsive to community preferences, needs, and values regarding health and health care	Measures of patient satisfaction with health care services	Measures of the extent to which community priorities have been identified and incorporated into community health improvement and investment decisions Measures of satisfaction with various aspects of the community that influence health, including availability of parks and recreational facilities, levels of environmental hazards (e.g., air and water quality), and investments in health care	Establishment of training programs for health care professionals to enhance communication skills and interactions with patients Assurance of the availability of language translation and other services that are responsive to the needs of the patient population being served	Establishment of tailored population health programs for minority populations, which are responsive to ethnic, cultural, and language issues Redesign of community space to encourage biking and walking

receiving appropriate services. Many factors can contribute to delays, for example, a scarcity of providers, the need for patients to travel long distances to provider sites, and lack of public transportation. Measures of delivery system timeliness include average waiting time for routine care and elective procedures and response time for emergency medical services.

At the population level, timeliness captures a different dimension of performance—early intervention to prevent or delay the onset and progression of disease. Examples of interventions that might improve timeliness are the expansion of health insurance coverage and safety net programs to improve access to preventive and primary care services, and communitywide educational programs aimed at parents of young children to encourage proper diet and exercise at the earliest possible age. Table 2-4 lists some illustrative strategies for improving timeliness.

Efficiency

From a population health perspective, efficiency includes two components:

- The avoidance of waste (including waste of equipment, supplies, ideas, and energy) in the delivery of population health services
- The efficient allocation of community resources and assets to population health programs to maximize health impact for the community

The second of these components is to a great extent what the committee is hoping to achieve through this integrated framework. Table 2-5 provides examples of efficiency improvement strategies.

Equity

From a population perspective, equity means all community residents have access to high-quality care that meets population-based health needs, and all community residents have the opportunity to live in an environment that promotes health (see Table 2-6). This aim implies that all Americans, whether living in rural or urban areas, have equitable access, quality, and financing of health care. Population-level measures of equity include percent of residents identifying a usual source of care and rates of exposure to environmental hazards for various racial and ethnic subpopulations. Community-level interventions to improve equity might include public policy

TABLE 2-4 Personal Health Care System and Community-Level Interventions: Illustrative Examples for Timeliness

Definition		Measures		Interventions	
Personal Health Focus	Population Health Focus	Personal Health Care System	Community Level	Personal Health Care System	Community Level
Reduce waits and sometimes harmful delays for both those who receive and those who give care	Ensure early intervention to prevent or delay the onset and progression of disease	Measures of timely receipt of services for patients (e.g., average wait times for routine care and elective procedures) Response time for emergency services	Population-based measures of obesity and diabetes (by stage of illness) by population age group	Enhanced hospital and office scheduling systems and redesign of care processes to improve patient flow Enhanced recruitment and retention of providers of emergency services	Community-level education programs on the importance of nutrition and exercise, aimed at parents of young children Public policy to encourage nutritious meals and exercise programs in schools

TABLE 2-5 Personal Health Care System and Community-Level Interventions: Illustrative Examples for Efficiency

Definition		Measures		Interventions	
Personal Health Focus	Population Health Focus	Personal Health Care System	Community Level	Personal Health Care System	Community Level
Avoid waste, including waste of equipment, supplies, ideas, and energy, in the delivery of personal health care services	Avoid waste, including waste of equipment, supplies, ideas, and energy, in the delivery of population health services	Measures of clinical efficiency (e.g., rates of use of evidence-based practices)	Tobacco cessation rates associated with per capita expenditures on communitywide smoking cessation programs	Dissemination of best practices regarding outpatient and inpatient workflow efficiency	Public reporting of population-based measures of health care use
	Seek efficient allocation of community resources and assets to personal and population health services to maximize health impact for the community	Measures of production efficiency (e.g., average annual health care costs for care of a patient with diabetes)	Measures of average days lost from work or school due to preventable illness per resident	Financial incentives to providers to reward adherence to protocols and coordination of care	Development of public policy that encourages (through financial and other incentives) a balance between personal health care and community health improvement programs
		Measures of clinician time spent on paperwork		Finance strategies that allow for more flexible integration of services (e.g., behavioral health, long-term care)	
		Measures of service duplication (e.g., ordering of redundant tests)		Investment in electronic health records	

TABLE 2-6 Personal Health Care System and Community-Level Interventions: Illustrative Examples for Equity

Definition		Measures		Interventions	
Personal Health Focus	Population Health Focus	Personal Health Care System	Community Level	Personal Health Care System	Community Level
Provide care that does not vary in quality because of personal characteristics, such as gender, ethnicity, geographic location, and socioeconomic status	Provide rural community residents with access to high-quality care that meets population-based health needs	Patient perceptions of the acceptability of services, stratified by race, ethnicity, religion, and other relevant subgroups	Measures of health care access and use across subpopulations and geographic areas	Sponsoring of cultural competency training for health care professionals	Development of public policy that encourages (through financial and other incentives) a geographic balance of health care providers
	Provide all community residents with an environment that promotes health (e.g., smoke-free public establishments)	Measures of differences in the appropriateness of services provided to patients of different racial and ethnic backgrounds	Rates of exposure to environmental hazards (e.g., lead poisoning) by race, ethnicity, and zip code		Cultivation of strong leadership and public–private partnerships (between the health care sector and other community stakeholders) to raise awareness of environmental forces that have a disproportionate impact on the health of minorities

and communitywide planning to locate providers in nearby underserved areas, and public programs to address environmental hazards that have a disproportionate impact on minorities.

Leadership and Collaboration

In light of the fundamental changes under way in health care, there is a critical need for strong leadership in rural communities. A great deal of attention has been focused on external forces that shape a community's health care system, such as public and private purchasers' payment policies, state practice regulations, and government programs and policies in support of health professions education. These external forces are important, but community-based efforts and solutions must play a role as well (Amundson, 1993).

Strong leadership will be needed within health care institutions (e.g., hospital CEOs and board members) and the professional community to redesign the care delivery system to achieve the six aims set forth in the *Quality Chasm* report (IOM, 2001) (see Chapter 1). Addressing safety and quality concerns in hospital, ambulatory, and other settings requires developing a new culture and making changes in organizational management and care processes. The development of models of care delivery that better meet the needs of a chronically ill population will necessitate fostering stronger collaborative relationships among (1) the various health professionals that constitute the care team, (2) the various institutions and provider settings within a rural community that make up the delivery system, and (3) the providers within a rural community and other essential providers outside the community (e.g., tertiary care centers, telemedicine specialty providers).

Strong leadership will also be needed to engage the broader rural community in health and health care issues. Efforts to strengthen what are often fragile delivery systems in rural areas will be more successful to the extent that they engage key stakeholders in a community (e.g., employers, schools, local government) (Amundson, 1993). Addressing population health needs and providing ongoing support for those with chronic illnesses will also necessitate collaboration with social services and faith-based organizations. Health care institutions will need to partner with schools, local media, libraries, and other organizations in their efforts to raise population health literacy. Lastly, fundamental reform of the personal and population health systems will necessitate developing innovative approaches to the financing and delivery of health services.

Every rural community needs its own health care leadership to participate in strategic planning, oversee the management of services delivered locally, and ensure accountability to local needs (Calico et al., 2003). Committed leadership of senior clinicians and administrators is key to the institutional and environment changes necessary to achieve improved quality of care and patient safety—a task that may at the same time be more difficult in rural areas because of personal connections that amplify feelings of blame for errors and easier because of the fewer layers of bureaucracy in rural health care delivery (Wakefield, 2002).

The W. K. Kellogg Foundation's Leadership for Community Change program offers an example of how community-based rural leaders can be cultivated. Begun in 2003, this program will work closely with local organizations at six rural and urban sites around the country to recruit a cohort of fellows (25 per site) who will participate in a mix of classroom training, mentoring, and networking at the national level over a period of 2 years (W. K. Kellogg Foundation, 2004). The program emphasizes the training of leaders already in place in their communities, rather than the identification and grooming of potential leaders from outside of the community, thus strengthening existing local resources.

Future leaders of rural health systems might also be cultivated through formal educational programs that broaden young health professionals' skills and knowledge of leadership competencies, health care organization and management, community planning and collaboration, epidemiology, and social and environmental services (Wheat et al., 2001). One approach that should be considered is the development of combined degree programs in public health and one of the clinical professions (e.g., medicine, pharmacy, nursing) that incorporate experiential learning opportunities in rural communities.

Recognizing the need for stronger leadership throughout the health care system, the National Center for Healthcare Leadership (NCHL) was established in 2001 (NCHL, 2003). With support from The Robert Wood Johnson Foundation and the W. K. Kellogg Foundation, NCHL's transformational leadership project has identified core competencies for health care management to ensure that management leadership is available to meet the needs of the health care sector, and has established an Advanced Learning Institute. Consideration should be given to establishing a learning collaborative for rural communities that could apply and build upon the work of NCHL and others.

CONCLUSIONS AND RECOMMENDATIONS

Rural communities, like much of America, face significant challenges in closing the quality gaps in both health care and population health status. In rural areas in particular, critical precursors to providing quality care are often in short supply. Many rural communities have long had difficulty attracting and retaining clinicians because of concerns about isolation, limited health facilities, or limited employment and education opportunities for their families. Health care systems in rural areas tend to be financially fragile (see Chapter 5), with some services, such as mental health and substance abuse, being critically underfunded. The human and technological infrastructures of rural health care are generally inadequate to support the quality improvement ambitions of rural communities and health care systems (see Chapters 4 and 6, respectively).

Rural America faces sizable challenges in improving population health behaviors. Obesity, for example, is a major health issue for many rural communities, as is the case in many urban communities. Unless actions are taken now to improve health behaviors, the future burden of chronic disease in many rural communities will be enormous. In agricultural and mining communities, unintentional work-related injuries are a serious concern. It is critical, therefore, that existing and new resources aimed at improving rural health and health care be deployed strategically to maximize the cost-effectiveness of those investments, recognizing both the need to improve the quality of individual-level care and the desire to improve the health of rural communities and populations.

In many respects, rural communities and areas have been on the margins of national health care quality discussions. Given the characteristics of rural environments, there is a need for critical analysis of the relevance of urban-derived quality efforts. This analysis should include reassessing, refining, and adapting some applications while also identifying new approaches tailored to rural communities. A roadmap for applying the quality agenda evolving at a national level to sparsely populated areas is needed. The goals of making care safe, effective, patient-centered, timely, efficient, and equitable for rural and frontier communities necessitate designing systems that build on the human and capital resources available in rural America. The committee has proposed using a decision-making framework that (1) links decisions within the personal health care delivery system more closely to the achievement of population health priorities, and (2) involves explicitly considering both personal and population-level interventions when making investment decisions. This framework is intended to provide a guide for health system reform and action in rural areas, and perhaps urban areas as well. Although this chapter has provided illustrative examples of how the framework can be applied, much work remains to be done in determining strategic health priorities in rural America and in identifying and evaluating alternative interventions at the personal health care and population levels.

> *Key Finding 1. A wide range of interventions are available to improve health and health care in rural America, but priorities for implementation are not yet clear. The Health Resources and Services Administration is the obvious agency to take the lead in setting priorities, in collaboration with other federal agencies, such as the Agency for Healthcare Research and Quality and the Centers for Disease Control and Prevention, as well as with rural stakeholders. This would entail systematically cataloguing and evaluating the potential of interventions to improve health care quality and population health in rural communities.*

As discussed in Chapter 1, the IOM report *Fostering Rapid Advances in Health Care: Learning from System Demonstrations* (IOM, 2003b) suggests a set of bottom-up strategies for health system reform that would enable states and/or communities (or "market areas") to mount demonstrations to test alternative strategies for creating a twenty-first century health care system. Not surprisingly, most innovations in health care, including those in quality improvement and safety, emerge from and are designed for urban-based, usually academically based, health centers. Yet application of these strategies in rural environments can be difficult if not impossible. These strategies and approaches need to be modified to fit the realities of the rural health care environment, and rural-derived quality innovation needs to be strengthened and supported.

The committee believes not only that rural communities must participate in such demonstrations, but also that, because of their smaller scale, more cohesive community structures, and other unique characteristics, rural areas and health systems offer an excellent opportunity to undertake and evaluate significant health system reform initiatives. The committee recognizes the challenges of attempting to develop communitywide programs that encompass and integrate population and personal health services (Kindig and Stoddart, 2003). But unless one assumes unlimited future investments in health care, prioritizing investments in the rural health care system will be critical.

> **Recommendation 1. Congress should provide the appropriate authority and resources to the Department of Health and Human Services to support comprehensive health system reform demonstrations in five rural communities. These demonstrations should evaluate alter-**

native models for achieving greater integration of personal and population health services and innovative approaches to the financing and delivery of health services, with the goal of meeting the six quality aims of the *Quality Chasm* report. The Agency for Healthcare Research and Quality, working collaboratively with the Health Resources and Services Administration, should ensure that the lessons learned from these demonstrations are disseminated to other communities, both urban and rural.

These demonstration projects would involve the establishment of collaborative structures, community-based prioritization of potential investments in health, and the development of communitywide population health programs. As discussed in Chapter 3, there will be a need for communitywide quality measurement and monitoring systems that include measures of both population health and the quality of care provided through the health care delivery system. Some of these demonstrations may well involve the implementation of new payment models, for example, a capitation payment approach administered at the community level, encompassing financing for both population and personal health. Additional work is needed to identify alternative payment models that are consistent with the committee's integrated approach, and to describe how such models might be tested through demonstrations in rural communities.

Residents of rural America are diverse, but one thing they generally do have in common is a strong sense of attachment to their community. This community orientation, combined with the smaller scale of rural health, human services, and community systems, may afford rural communities an opportunity to demonstrate more rapidly the vision of balancing and integrating the needs of personal health care with broader communitywide initiatives that target the entire population (IOM, 2003b).

Efforts should also be made to build stronger rural communities that mobilize all types of institutions (e.g., health care, educational, social, and faith-based) to both augment and support the contributions of health professionals. As discussed above, to achieve the greatest improvement across all six quality aims, rural communities will need to focus greater attention and resources on improving population health. Doing so will necessitate building coalitions. Some coalitions will involve stakeholders from within the health care sector; for example, the providers in a community might pool resources to sponsor a communitywide education program aimed at the prevention and early diagnosis and treatment of diabetes. Other coalitions will engage stakeholders outside the traditional health care sector in efforts to improve population health; for example, efforts to reduce obesity in children might include outreach to school leaders to encourage the provision of more nutritious lunches and snacks. For the most part, the leadership for both types of efforts will need to come from the health sector. Too often today, practicing health professionals do not feel they have the skills or interests to offer sustained leadership in these domains.

> *Key Finding 2. Rural communities engaged in health system redesign would likely benefit from leadership training programs. Such training programs could be provided by the Agency for Healthcare Research and Quality and the Office of Rural Health Policy working collaboratively with private- and public-sector organizations involved in leadership development, such as the National Council for Healthcare Leadership and the W. K. Kellogg Foundation's Leadership for Community Change Program.*

AHRQ and the Office of Rural Health Policy should work together to sponsor leadership training programs in rural areas. Consideration should also be given to collaborating with private-sector groups engaged in leadership development, such as the National Council for Healthcare Leadership and the W. K. Kellogg Foundation's Leadership for Community Change Program.

REFERENCES

AHRQ (Agency for Healthcare Research and Quality). 2004. *Medical Errors and Patient Safety*. [Online]. Available: http://www.ahrq.gov/qual/errorsix.htm [accessed September 29, 2004].

Amundson B. 1993. Myth and reality in the rural health service crisis: Facing up to community responsibilities. *Journal of Rural Health* 9(3):176–187.

Anderson GF, Hussey PS. 2001. Comparing health system performance in OECD countries. *Health Affairs* 20(3):219–232.

Baldwin LM, MacLehose RF, Hart G, Beaver SK, Every N, Chan L. 2004. Quality of care for acute myocardial infarction in rural and urban U.S. hospitals. *Journal of Rural Health* 20(2):99–108.

Calico F, Dillard C, Moscovice I, Wakefield M. 2003. A framework and action agenda for quality improvement in rural health care. *Journal of Rural Health* 19(3):226–232.

Coburn A, Wakefield M, Casey M, Moscovice I, Payne S, Loux S. Forthcoming. Assuring rural hospital patient safety: What should the priorities be? *Journal of Rural Health* 20(4):314–326.

Cromartie J. 2002. Nonmetro migration continues downward trend. *Rural America* 17(4):70–73.

Detmer DE, Singleton PD, Macleod A, Wait S, Taylor M, Ridwell J. 2003 (March). *The Informed Patient: Study Report.* Cambridge, UK: Judge Institute of Management, Cambridge University Health.

Gamm L, Hutchison L, Bellamy G, Dabney B. 2002. Rural healthy people 2010: Identifying rural health priorities and models for practice. *Journal of Rural Health* 18(1):9–14.

Grossman DC, Kim A, Macdonald SC, Klein P, Copass MK, Maier RV. 1997. Urban-rural differences in prehospital care of major trauma. *Journal of Trauma* 42(4):723–729.

Gurwitz JH, Field TS, Avorn J, McCormick D, Jain S, Eckler M, Benser M, Edmondson AC, Bates DW. 2000. Incidence and preventability of adverse drug events in nursing homes. *American Journal of Medicine* 109(2):87–94.

Gurwitz JH, Field TS, Harrold LR, Rothchild J, Debellis K, Seger AC, Cadoret C, Fish LS, Garber L, Kelleher M, Bates DW. 2003. Incidence and preventability of adverse drug events among older persons in the ambulatory setting. *Journal of the American Medical Association* 289(9):1107–1116.

Hillemeier MM, Lynch J, Harper S, Casper M. 2003. Measuring contextual characteristics for community health. *Health Services Research* 38(6):1645–1717.

HRSA (Health Resources and Services Administration, Bureau of Primary Care). 2004. *The Community Access Program.* [Online]. Available: http://bphc.hrsa.gov/cap/Default.htm [accessed September 14, 2004].

Hussey PS, Anderson GF, Osborn R, Feek C, McLaughlin V, Millar J, Epstein A. 2004. How does the quality of care compare in five countries? *Health Affairs* 23(3):89–99.

IOM (Institute of Medicine). 2000. *To Err Is Human: Building a Safer Health System.* Washington, DC: National Academy Press.

IOM. 2001. *Crossing the Quality Chasm: A New Health System for the 21st Century.* Washington, DC: National Academy Press.

IOM. 2002. *Care Without Coverage: Too Little Too Late.* Washington, DC: The National Academies Press.

IOM. 2003a. *Unequal Treatment: Confronting Racial and Ethnic Disparities in Health Care.* Washington, DC: The National Academies Press.

IOM. 2003b. *Fostering Rapid Advances in Health Care: Learning from System Demonstrations.* Washington, DC: The National Academies Press.

IOM. 2004. *Patient Safety: Achieving a New Standard for Care.* Washington, DC: The National Academies Press.

JCAHO (Joint Commission on the Accreditation of Healthcare Organizations). 2004 (January). *Special Report: Shared Visions—New Pathways.* [Online]. Available: http://www.jcaho.org/accredited+organizations/svnp/jcp-2004-january.pdf [accessed January 2004].

Jolliffe D. 2003. Nonmetro poverty: Assessing the effect of the 1990s. *Amber Waves* 1(4):30–33.

Kazandjian VA. 2003. *Accountability Through Measurement: A Global Healthcare Imperative.* Milwaukee, WI: ASQ Quality Press. Pp. 326–328.

Kindig D, Stoddart GL. 2003. What is population health? *American Journal of Public Health* 93(3):380–383.

LaLonde M. 1975. *A New Perspective on the Health of Canadians.* Ottawa, Canada: Ministry of National Health and Welfare.

Lorig KR, Sobel DS, Stewart AL, Brown BW Jr, Bandura A, Ritter P, Gonzalez VM, Laurent DD, Holman HR. 1999. Evidence suggesting that a chronic disease self-management program can improve health status while reducing hospitalization: A randomized trial. *Medical Care* 37(1):5–14.

Maynard C, Every NR, Chapko MK, Ritchie JL. 2000. Outcomes of coronary angioplasty procedures performed in rural hospitals. *American Journal of Medicine* 108(9):748–750.

McGinnis MJ, Williams-Russo P, Knickman JR. 2002. The case for more active policy attention to health promotion. *Health Affairs* 21:78–93.

McGlynn EA, Asch SM, Adams J, Keesey J, Hicks J, DeCristofaro A, Kerr EA. 2003. The quality of health care delivered to adults in the United States. *New England Journal of Medicine* 348(26):2635–2645.

Morrisey MA, Ohsfelt RL, Johnson V, Treat R. 1995. Rural emergency medical services: Patients, destinations, times, and services. *Journal of Rural Health* 11(4):286–294.

NCHL (National Center of Health Care Leadership). 2003. *2003 Annual Report.* Chicago, IL: National Center for Healthcare Leadership.

NCHS (National Center for Health Statistics). 2001. *Health, United States, 2001 with Urban and Rural Health Chartbook.* Washington, DC: U.S. Department of Health and Human Services.

Nesbitt TS, Yellowlees PM, Hogarth M, Hilty DM. 2004 (March). *Rural Health Care in the Digital Age: The Role of Information and Telecommunications Technologies in the Future of Rural Health.* Commissioned Paper for the IOM Committee on the Future of Rural Health Care. Washington, DC.

NQF (The National Quality Forum). 2003. *Safe Practices for Better Healthcare: A Consensus Report.* Washington, DC: NQF.

Ormond B, Zuckerman S, Lhila A. May 2000. *Rural/Urban Differences in Health Care Are Not Uniform Across States.* Washington, DC: The Urban Institute.

Pol LG, Rouse J, Zyzanski S, Rasmussen D, Crabtree B. 2001. Rural, urban, and suburban comparisons of preventive services in family practice clinics. *Journal of Rural Health* 17(2):114–121.

Reiber GM, Benzie D, McMahon S. 1996. Why patients bypass rural health care centers. *Minnesota Medicine* 79:46–50.

Reinhardt UE, Hussey PS, Anderson GF. 2004. U.S. health care spending in an international context. *Health Affairs* 23(3):10–25.

Romano PS, Geppert JJ, Davies S, Miller MR, Elixhauser A, McDonald KM. 2003. A national profile of patient safety in U.S. hospitals. *Health Affairs* 22(2):154–166.

Rosenblatt RA, Baldwin L, Chan L, Fordyce MA, Hirsch IB, Palmer JP, Wright GE, Hart LG. 2001. Improving the quality of outpatient care for older patients with diabetes: Lessons from a comparison of rural and urban communities. *Journal of Family Practice* 50(8):676–680.

Sackett DL, Rosenberg WM, Muir Gray JA, Haynes RB, Richardson WS. 1996. Evidence-based medicine: What it is and what it isn't. *British Medical Journal* 312:71–72.

Shojania KG, Duncan BW, McDonald KM, Wachter RM. 2002. Safe but sound: Patient safety meets evidence-based medicine. *Journal of the American Medical Association* 288(4):508–513.

Thomas EJ, Studdert DM, Newhouse JP, Zbar BI, Howard KM, Williams EJ, Brennan TA. 1999. Costs of medical injuries in Utah and Colorado. *Inquiry* 36:255–264.

W. K. Kellogg Foundation. 2004. *Kellogg Leadership for Community Change.* [Online]. Available: http://www.klccleadership.org [accessed July 16, 2004].

Wagner EH. 1998. Chronic disease management: What will it take to improve care for chronic illness? *Effective Clinical Practice* 1(1):2–4.

Wakefield M. 2002. Patient safety and medical errors: Implications for rural health care. *Journal of Legal Medicine* 23:43–56.

Wheat JR, Donham KJ, Simpson WM. 2001. Medical education for agricultural health and safety. *Journal of Agromedicine* 8(1):77–92.

Whitener L, McGranahan D. 2003. Rural America: Opportunities and challenges. *Amber Waves* 1(1):15–21.

WHO (World Health Organization). 2000. *World Health Report 2000.* Geneva, Switzerland: WHO.

Williamson JW, Fehlauer CS, Gaiennie J, Smith CB. 1991. Assessing quality of ambulatory care: A comparative analysis in rural versus tertiary general medical clinics. *Quality Assurance Utilization Review* 6(1):8–15.

Wisconsin Medical Society. 2002–2003. *Policy Compendium 2002–2003.* [Online]. Available: http://www.wisconsinmedicalsociety.org/health_policy/COMP/rur.cfm [accessed July 2004].

3

Quality Improvement Activities in Rural Areas

SUMMARY

Health care quality is highly variable and falls far short of what it should be in all environments (see Chapter 2). To improve quality, rural providers, like their urban counterparts, must adopt a comprehensive approach to quality improvement. This approach needs to encompass clinical knowledge and the tools necessary to apply this knowledge to practice, including practice guidelines and computer-aided decision support, standardized performance measures, performance measurement and data feedback capabilities, and quality improvement processes and resources. This chapter examines each of these capabilities, with emphasis on their current state of development in rural health systems and steps that might be taken to enhance quality improvement in rural communities.

It should be noted that this chapter focuses on quality improvement processes and activities, while Chapter 6 addresses information and communications technology infrastructure. These two issues are intricately related: electronic health records, including computerized decision support and web-based communication, offer the potential to vastly improve the effectiveness and efficiency of quality improvement processes and activities.

Serious shortcomings in the quality of care need to be addressed in both rural and urban communities. But confronting the same challenge does not imply the same solution. As discussed earlier, rural and urban areas vary in their beliefs, customs, practices, and social behaviors, as well as in the availability of human and technological resources. The quality aims are the same—to provide care that is safe, effective, patient-centered, timely, efficient, and equitable—but the means of achieving these aims may differ.

In addressing the quality challenge, rural communities must build on their strengths. Ironically, these strengths stem directly from the major weakness of delivering care in rural areas—the scarcity of resources and providers. In rural communities where the need for services far exceeds the available supply, providers may be more willing and able to work together and with their patients and communities to develop a community health system that best meets the needs of individual patients and the entire population.

This chapter first sets forth the key components of a health care quality improvement program, and suggests how these components apply in particular to the rural context. The second section reviews the current state of quality improvement efforts in rural areas. The final section presents conclusions and recommendations.

KEY COMPONENTS OF A COMPREHENSIVE QUALITY IMPROVEMENT PROGRAM

The quality infrastructure needed to support quality improvement involves both national and regional/local components. Successful efforts require leadership, cultural change in organizations, and human resources and technical support. In particular, to achieve the six quality aims cited above (and in Chapter 1), rural communities must establish comprehensive quality improvement programs that include five key components (see Box 3-1). It is important to emphasize that all of these components must be supported by information and communications technology (ICT), including electronic health records (EHRs) and web-based communication.

Knowledge of the Science of Quality and Safety Improvement

Quality improvement is an ongoing process that draws on a multidisciplinary knowledge base (i.e., statistics, epidemiology, engineering, human factors analysis) and employs many tools (e.g., control charts, root-cause analysis of adverse events) to identify and understand shortcomings and redesign care processes. Knowledge of the science of quality and safety im-

BOX 3-1
Key Components of a Comprehensive
Quality Improvement Program

Any comprehensive quality improvement program must encompass five key components:

- Knowledge of the science of quality and safety improvement
- Clinical knowledge and the tools needed to apply this knowledge, especially practice guidelines, protocols, and computer-aided decision support
- Standardized performance measures
- Performance measurement and data feedback capabilities
- Quality improvement processes and resources

Information and communications technology, including electronic health records and web-based communication, provides an essential foundation for all of these components.

SOURCE: Adapted from Brent James, IOM Workshop Presentation, 2003.

provement is critical to the development of a culture within the health care system and the health care community overall that values quality and embraces opportunities to improve it. As discussed in Chapter 4, this knowledge base is important to three groups of stakeholders: health care leaders, health care professionals, and health care consumers. An understanding of quality and safety (including the current state of quality, as well as quality improvement theory and tools) is essential to community leaders engaged in health system reform. Moreover, quality improvement knowledge—including methods of identifying errors and hazards in care; safety design principles, such as standardization and simplification; quality measurement in terms of structure, process, and outcomes; and methods of designing and testing interventions to improve care processes—is a core competency that all health care professionals should possess (IOM, 2003). Also, rural residents need to understand quality and safety issues if they are to work collaboratively with clinicians to improve care and engage in self-management of their health and health care (Detmer et al., 2003).

Clinical Knowledge and Associated Tools

Like their urban counterparts, rural communities need access to clinical knowledge and the tools needed to apply this knowledge to practice. Three types of tools are particularly important—practice guidelines, protocols, and computer-aided decision support. Physicians, nurses, pharmacists, and other clinicians struggle to stay abreast of scientific knowledge. Clinicians can more easily apply the large body of scientific knowledge when it has been translated into practice guidelines by professional groups. To apply scientific knowledge and practice guidelines in rural communities, some additional work is required. Local protocols, (i.e., stepwise instructions to guide local care delivery) must be developed that reflect the specific challenges of rural communities. For example, when highly specialized care is needed (e.g., treatment of trauma due to brain injury), the protocol for a rural community would likely draw upon practice guidelines for head injuries and stabilization and transfer of the patient to a tertiary center. Moreover, to be useful to laypersons in making decisions about their health behaviors and health care, scientific knowledge must be made available in ways that reflect the health literacy of the population, which is a function of many factors, including education, language ability, and culture (see Chapter 4). Finally, the ability of clinicians and patients to apply knowledge and guidelines when making health-related decisions may be enhanced when the knowledge and guidelines are used to develop reminder systems (e.g., computerized reminders to patients and their clinicians that patients are due for an annual pap smear) and alerts (e.g., notice that the patient is about to be prescribed a medication that is contraindicated). As discussed in Chapter 6, the development of EHRs opens up many possibilities to incorporate a wide array of prompts and alerts into clinical practice that draw upon the science base and the full set of patient data available in the EHR.

Standardized Performance Measures

An appropriate set of standardized performance measures is needed to assess whether performance is consistent with the evidence base and results in improved care processes and patient outcomes. The use of standardized measures makes it possible to compare providers within and across geographic areas for purposes of identifying best practices.

Recent years have seen tremendous growth in the use of standardized measurement sets for health plans, hospitals, ambulatory care, nursing homes, and home health care. There are standardized measure sets that are specific to particular clinical conditions and surgical procedures (e.g., diabetes, thoracic surgery); that assess the quality of nursing care; that assess how well certain core processes are performed (e.g., care coordination); and that rely on patient reports and assessments of care.

Rural communities stand to benefit a great deal from the development of these quality measurement tools. Many of the standardized measures included in leading measure sets are applicable to both rural and urban settings. But there are instances where measure sets need to be adapted to be most useful in rural settings, and there are specific implementation challenges that arise frequently in rural settings as well. Casey and Moscovice (2004) identify specific aspects of the rural context that must be considered when applying standardized measure sets for use in rural hospitals:

• *Small size*—Small rural provider settings often lack adequate numbers of patients with particular conditions or requiring specific procedures to construct reliable measures.

• *A scarcer and more diverse resource context*—Differing resource contexts will lead to different care processes in rural and urban hospitals. For example, a pharmacist is most typically not available 24 hours a day in rural hospitals and community-based pharmacies, necessitating alternative arrangements, such as preparation of certain medications by nursing staff in the hospital or use of an "on call" pharmacist in the community.

• *First-contact and linking role*—An important role for many rural hospitals is triage and the stabilization and transfer of emergency cases. Rural measurement sets should include measures for assessing how well this function is performed.

• *Community hub*—Rural hospitals are central and influential organizations in their communities; in many rural communities, the hospital is the largest employer in town. Many rural hospitals are assuming a coordinating role to support the development of more integrated community-based care systems. The assumption of this role affords an opportunity to include measures of population health and communitywide service integration in rural measurement sets.

This last point, the community hub role, deserves special emphasis. In Chapter 2 of this report, the committee presents an integrated framework for addressing population and personal health care needs, and proposes the conduct of comprehensive health reform demonstrations in five rural communities. Rural communities pursuing such efforts will need communitywide measurement and monitoring systems that include both population-level measures and measures at the level of the health care delivery system. Also, as discussed in Chapter 5, rural communities incorporating pay-for-performance programs or alternative payment models into a demonstration project may well choose to tie payment incentives to the achievement of population and personal health goals.

Efforts are already under way to identify and adapt leading measure sets for application in rural provider sites (Casey and Moscovice, 2004). In particular, the American Hospital Association is currently developing a rural version of the measure sets for myocardial infarction, heart failure, and pneumonia that are used in the National Voluntary Hospital Reporting Initiative (Personal communication, N. Foster, July 9, 2004). For example, since rural hospitals stabilize and transfer patients more frequently than do urban hospitals, the discharge measures need to be adjusted to better reflect and ensure quality of care in patient transfers.

Performance Measurement and Data Feedback Capabilities

Local health systems must have performance measurement systems capable of monitoring progress across a well-balanced set of standardized performance measures and providing timely feedback to administrative and clinical staff (e.g., comparative reports). At present, most performance measurement and improvement activities rely on data abstracted from paper medical records, culled from administrative datasets, or in some cases maintained in disease registries. While these have historically been the most important data sources and should be fully exploited by quality improvement programs, they have serious limitations. Administrative files and registries lack the comprehensive and clinically rich data necessary to address many important aspects of performance and to adjust for differences such as severity of illness. Abstraction of paper medical records is a slow and resource-intensive process. The same ICT infrastructure (see Chapter 6) that is needed to provide real-time computer-aided decision support to providers can support the performance measurement monitoring process.

Quality Improvement Processes and Resources

Well-thought-out quality improvement processes with adequate human and technical resources are essential to accomplishing the six quality aims.

Small hospitals and ambulatory practices often lack the resources needed to establish a robust quality improvement program. As noted above, small providers may also lack adequate numbers of patients with specific conditions to conduct certain types of analyses. One alternative is for rural communities to work together in a collaborative fashion to establish communitywide quality improvement programs. These programs might also pool data for all providers in the community and conduct population-based analyses. Another option is for individual rural providers to participate in collaborative efforts sponsored by outside organizations, such as the Institute for Healthcare Improvement or a Medicare Quality Improvement Organization (QIO).

CURRENT STATE OF QUALITY IMPROVEMENT EFFORTS IN RURAL AREAS

Many rural and urban providers have been slow to adopt state-of-the-art quality improvement techniques. Rural providers in particular have found it difficult to invest in quality improvement because of their small scale and low operating margins (see Chapter 5 and Appendix C). Also, as discussed below, some national quality improvement efforts, designed to meet the needs of the majority of providers, are a poor fit for rural settings. In recent years, some targeted support has been provided for rural quality improvement programs, and there are early signs that these investments are paying off.

Quality Improvement Organizations

The Centers for Medicare and Medicaid Services (CMS) contracts with 53 QIOs to offer providers assistance with quality improvement (CMS, 2003b). QIOs engage in a variety of activities, including many disease-specific quality measurement and improvement projects and education and complaint resolution for beneficiaries. More recently, QIOs have assumed some responsibility for public reporting of comparative performance data.

Concern has been raised that rural providers do not receive their fair share of QIO assistance (MedPAC, 2001; NACRHHS, 2001, 2003). Prior to 2002, QIOs operating on a fixed budget under contract with CMS had little incentive to focus attention on small rural providers because they were evaluated on the basis of their ability to reach a large proportion of the population or to improve statewide averages on a range of quality indicators (CMS,

2003b). Quality improvement activities focused on large urban hospitals are more likely to impact a sizable segment of the population and/or to result in improved state averages on quality indicators, and have the added advantage of being geographically more accessible to QIO staff.

In 2002, CMS modified the scope of work for QIOs to include a specific subtask requiring them to improve care for rural beneficiaries or address racial and ethnic disparities in care (CMS, 2003a). However, the evaluation criteria for QIOs still reward improvements in statewide averages on performance indicators. Many QIOs have likely chosen to satisfy the requirements of this subtask by addressing racial or ethnic disparities in urban areas, again because those areas are more geographically accessible to QIO staff and are home to large health care organizations that have a greater impact on statewide performance.

The American Health Quality Association, a membership association representing QIOs, reports that nearly 20 state QIOs are working with critical access hospitals and ambulatory care providers in rural areas (Personal communication, D. G. Schulke, March 18, 2004). Another 17 states, having 20 percent or more of their population residing in rural areas, have no formal rural health project (Personal communication, D. G. Schulke, September 17, 2003).

Although the QIO program as a whole focuses too little attention on rural providers, some QIOs, most notably those in states with large rural populations, are extensively involved in rural quality improvement. For example, Qualis Health in Idaho, in collaboration with the Idaho Hospital Association and the Idaho Department of Health and Welfare, is sponsoring a project for critical access hospitals in Idaho (AHQA, 2004). Stratis Health, the Minnesota QIO, is also working with critical access hospitals on a quality collaborative focused initially on heart failure, smoking cessation, and inpatient influenza and pneumococcal immunizations, with the long-term goal of developing quality initiatives in all clinical areas (Stratis Health, 2004).

One option for addressing this ongoing concern is to decouple the QIOs' rural health work from their work on disparities in care by creating separate subtasks for each. This approach is recommended by the National Advisory Committee on Rural Health and Human Services in its recent report to the Secretary of Health and Human Services (NACRHHS, 2003). The American Health Quality Association also supports the creation of separate subtasks, but has proposed that QIOs with either very small or very large rural populations be able to opt out of the rural subtask (Personal communication, D. G. Schulke, September 17, 2003). QIOs with very small rural populations would be required to work with other stakeholders to try to address the needs of rural beneficiaries. In states with very large rural populations, a separate rural subtask would be redundant, since these states are already focusing a large proportion of their resources on rural areas as a means of improving statewide averages on quality indicators.

The committee supports the creation of separate subtasks for rural disparities and for racial and ethnic disparities. Inequities in health, health care, and quality improvement in both areas need to be addressed.

Concern has also been raised that many QIOs, given their limited focus on rural areas, lack the knowledge, experience, and tools necessary to offer technical assistance to rural providers. CMS has addressed the need for specialized knowledge and expertise in other areas through the creation of Quality Improvement Organization Support Centers (QIOSCs). One option for dealing with this issue would be to create a QIOSC specific to rural health, which could play a lead role in the development of rural-specific quality measures, educational programs, and improvement tools and approaches. This QIOSC should build on the collaborative effort already under way between the QIOs in Minnesota and Utah/Nevada to field test a set of rural-relevant hospital quality measures.

Public Reporting Programs

In recent years, both the public and private sectors have launched numerous public reporting initiatives. The Department of Health and Human Services has reporting initiatives focused on the nation as a whole and on states and on health plans and providers (USDHHS, 2001). In addition, many private-sector reporting efforts are sponsored by purchasers, providers, and accreditation entities. Of particular importance are the efforts of The Leapfrog Group, whose members include 150 public- and private-sector organizations that provide health benefits. Following is a brief summary of some of the more significant efforts under way:

- *National Healthcare Quality Report (NHQR)*—In December 2003, the Agency for Healthcare Research and Quality (AHRQ) released the first NHQR, providing the country with a snapshot of quality for the nation as a whole (AHRQ, 2003b). The report includes quality measures pertaining to each of the six quality aims, as well as measures applicable to many leading chronic conditions. A companion report, the *National Disparities Report*, provides national data specific to rural areas for many of the quality measures associated with effectiveness, patient safety, and timeliness of care, as well as data associated with disparities in access to care among rural residents (AHRQ, 2003a).

• *Medicare Compare*—Starting in 1999, CMS began producing comparative performance reports for providers that participate in the Medicare program. The reports are available online through links to the Medicare Compare databases for each provider type. The series now includes *Medicare Health Plan Compare*,[1] *Dialysis Facility Compare, Nursing Home Compare*, and *Home Health Compare* (CMS, 2004a). *Hospital Compare*, to be added in early 2005, is based on voluntary reporting, but the number of participating hospitals is expected to grow rapidly since participation is required for hospitals to receive the full "market basket" payment update under the Prospective Payment System (Public Law 108-173, Section 501) (CMS, 2004b). Since many rural hospitals (i.e., critical access hospitals) are not paid under the Prospective Payment System, they do not have the same incentives to report data publicly. Some rural hospitals have chosen to participate, but overall participation rates will likely be lower for rural than for urban hospitals.

• *The Leapfrog Group*—In June 2001, The Leapfrog Group began requesting information from hospitals on an initial set of three safety practices (i.e., leaps): use of computerized physician order entry, evidence-based hospital referral (i.e., referral of patients with certain complex medical procedures to high-volume hospitals), and staffing of intensive care units with doctors who have specialized critical care training (see www.leapfroggroup. org/FactSheets/ LF_FactSheet.pdf). In April 2004, Leapfrog added a fourth leap consisting of 30 safe practices (e.g., standardized methods for labeling, packaging, and storing medications; standardized protocols to prevent the occurrence of wrong-site or wrong-patient procedures) identified by the National Quality Forum (NQF, 2003). Leapfrog formally requested data on the first three leaps from urban and suburban hospitals in 24 regions. With the addition of the new safe practices leap, rural hospitals will be encouraged to submit quality data to Leapfrog for the first time.

---

[1] Medicare Health Plan Compare also is referred to as Medicare Personal Plan Finder with links for Medicare Advantage Data and Medigap Data.

Public reporting has raised concern within the rural health care community. For the most part, this concern does not reflect an objection to the public reporting of performance data, but a belief that the current set of measures and reporting formats may not adequately consider the unique characteristics of rural health care delivery. As discussed above, many of the measures in leading measure sets will be appropriate for both urban and rural areas, but not all. In addition, there may be some measures of particular interest to rural communities that would not be of interest to urban. In designing public reports for rural areas, it will be important to identify when rural-to-rural comparisons are appropriate (e.g., emergency medical services response times, stabilization, and transfer). Also, public reports for rural communities as a whole (in contrast with provider-specific reports) may be the most useful and reliable, given the role of rural hospitals as a community hub and the methodological challenge of measurement at the provider level (i.e., small sample sizes). Community-based reports are also consistent with the committee's recommendation in Chapter 2 to focus attention on both population and personal health issues and to encourage communitywide collaboration. It would be advisable for CMS to work collaboratively with the rural community to identify the subset of measures for which rural/urban comparisons are appropriate and those for which comparisons should not be made, and to modify reporting formats to include explanatory material pertaining to rural/urban differences. Some consideration should also be given to producing a set of reports that present only rural/rural provider comparisons for certain measures, such as timeliness of emergency care (Moscovice, 2004).

The committee emphasizes that rural providers should not be excluded from public reporting initiatives. Public disclosure and eventually pay-for-performance payment methods (discussed in Chapter 5) are potentially powerful incentives for encouraging improvements in quality. Rural providers, like urban, will benefit from these external levers for change as long as the performance measures are reliable and valid and the comparative reports are fair. Further, the conspicuous absence of rural providers from public reports may have the unintended consequence of leading rural residents to assume that local providers are of lower quality than more distant providers, a conclusion not supported by the very limited evidence that is available for assessing differences in quality between rural and urban areas (see Chapter 2).

Targeted Rural Quality Programs

The Health Resources and Services Administration (HRSA) sponsors various quality programs aimed at rural populations. Although smaller in terms of resources than the quality efforts of AHRQ and CMS, these programs likely have a good deal of impact because they are specifically tailored to the needs of rural areas and sensitive to the constraints faced by rural providers. Three HRSA quality programs are discussed: the Rural Hospital Flexibility Grant Program (Flex), the Small Hospital Improvement Program (SHIP), and quality efforts focused on community health centers and rural health clinics. Also discussed are the quality requirements applicable to rural health clinics.

The Medicare Flex program was created in 1997 to provide additional financial support to small rural hospitals designated as critical access hospitals (see Appendix C). As of May 2004, 835 hospitals had been certified as critical access (FMT, 2004; Personal communication, S. Poley, July 7, 2004). HRSA's grant program provides grants to states to support activities in four areas: helping hospitals convert to critical access status, promoting rural health networks, integrating emergency services, and improving quality. In fiscal year 2004, HRSA awarded approximately $39.7 million in Flex grants to 45 states (Personal communication, J. Riggle, July 2, 2004). More than $4.3 million of this funding was used for quality improvement. One state, Montana, used these funds to create a statewide network among its critical access hospitals to collaborate on ongoing quality improvement activities by linking the network to the regional QIO; the network also supports collaboration on provider education, medical staff credentialing, and public reporting (NACRHHS, 2003).

In a telephone survey of more than 200 critical access hospitals conducted in 2000 and again in 2001, the responding hospitals reported significant increases in quality improvement activities, including continuing education programs for staff, data collection for staff feedback, systems to avoid/prevent errors, and medical error reporting policies (Moscovice et al., 2002). Many reported a redefinition of quality improvement processes, including greater formalization of policies and procedures and increased emphasis on quality improvement as compared with quality assurance. Many of the respondents reported collaboration with an affiliated hospital (47 percent), a QIO (45 percent), or a state hospital association (32 percent) on quality improvement activities. A more recent survey of a subset of critical access hospitals that had reported sizable improvements in their quality-related activities on earlier surveys revealed that four-fifths had implemented one or more clinical guidelines or protocols; two-thirds had enhanced improvement training for staff; and as a group these hospitals had implemented a wide range of quality improvement activities (e.g., projects focused on pneumonia, congestive heart failure, acute myocardial infarction, or stroke, as well as patient safety initiatives) (Moscovice et al., 1997).

In fiscal years 2002 and 2003, the SHIP program provided about $15 million each year to rural hospitals to support quality improvement projects and transitional efforts related to the new Medicare Prospective Payment System and the Health Insurance Portability and Accountability Act (NACRHHS, 2003). A total of 1,400 hospitals received small grants of less than $10,000 each in fiscal year 2002, and 28 percent of these hospitals used some or all of these funds for quality improvement.

The approximately 3,500 clinics participating in the rural health clinic program (discussed in Appendix C) must satisfy the requirements of CMS's quality assessment and performance improvement program (Balanced Budget Act of 1997, Public Law 105-133, Section 4205(b)). That program requires that rural health clinics evaluate clinical effectiveness (appropriateness, prevention), access to care (availability and accessibility, cultural competency, emergency interventions), patient satisfaction, and utilization of clinical services. A 2000 study of 40 rural health clinics in 10 different states found that the clinics' activities and capabilities varied widely, and few were prepared for implementation of the CMS program (Knott and Travers, 2002). The clinics indicated that technical assistance and staff training in all aspects of quality assurance would be needed to implement the program, along with more time and resources.

HRSA also provides support and technical assistance to the approximately 840 community health centers, a little more than one-half of which are located in rural areas (Personal communication, R. C. Lee, May 28, 2004). Technical assistance focuses on chronic care management, disease registries, the application of evidence-based practice guidelines, and quality measurement and improvement. Many community health centers have also been involved in a 6-year health disparities collaborative focused on diabetes (Chin et al., 2004).

Accreditation and Certification Programs

Accreditation and certification programs have played an important role in encouraging and facilitating the development of quality improvement programs and processes in the hospital sector. As a condition of participating in the Medicare program, hospitals must be either accredited by the Joint Commission on Accreditation of Healthcare Organizations (JCAHO) or federally certified.

Rural hospitals are less likely to seek accreditation through JCAHO than are urban hospitals. During the 10-year period from 1987 to 1996, the proportion of accredited urban hospitals remained fairly steady at 95 percent, while the proportion of accredited rural hospitals decreased from 62 to 58 percent (Brasure et al., 2000). In a survey of rural hospitals, 79 percent of respondents indicated that the cost of accreditation was a major deterrent, but there were other reasons as well: have no need or see no value (19 percent), standards unrealistic for small rural hospitals (16 percent), already surveyed by other agencies (11 percent), and other concerns regarding the JCAHO process (11 percent) (Brasure et al., 2000). In applying for accreditation, hospitals face two types of costs: survey fees paid to JCAHO (direct costs) and expenses associated with preparing for the survey, such as staff time or consultant fees (indirect costs). Recent changes in JCAHO's hospital accreditation program intended to streamline preparation should decrease the indirect costs somewhat (JCAHO, 2004). In addition, both JCAHO and the American Osteopathic Association have established special accreditation programs for critical access hospitals (Personal communication, K. Patton, July 7, 2004). It is too early to tell whether these changes will attract a sizable number of new entrants to the accreditation process.

As an alternative to accreditation, hospitals can be certified through a review process carried out by state governments. Most rural hospitals have chosen this route. There are no survey fees for certification. Unfortunately, state certification processes are highly variable, and state fiscal constraints often limit the frequency of reviews and the intensity of follow-up activities (Federal Register, 2002).

CONCLUSIONS AND RECOMMENDATIONS

Many aspects of an effective quality improvement infrastructure will be the same for rural and urban areas, but some aspects need to be customized to reflect key differences between rural and urban health systems and environments. In Chapter 1, the committee embraced the overarching objective that *rural Americans, like urban Americans, should have access to the full spectrum of high-quality, appropriate health care.* The committee also identified a set of guiding principles for operationalizing this overarching objective. These guiding principles recognize that there will be differences in the way rural and urban residents access some aspects of care. More specifically, urban areas are usually able to provide local access to the full spectrum of services needed by their population, while rural residents must travel to access certain specialized services. Most rural areas provide access to a core set of services, but are unable to generate an adequate volume of certain specialized services for providers to maintain their skills and financially support their practices (e.g., trauma centers, many subspecialty services). For rural residents who must travel to access certain services, some aspects of the care process are particularly important, such as, stabilization and transfer, and referral and coordination of services. In summary, for the majority of services and patient needs, rural and urban areas should be able to apply the same practice guidelines and performance measures, but for a limited number of areas, quality improvement tools will need to be customized to be relevant within a rural context. For benchmarking purposes, rural providers need access to comparative data, and for some types of measures (e.g., acute myocardial infarction, emergency care, stabilization and referral), rural-specific comparative data will be most relevant.

Rural communities must also have the flexibility and assistance needed to develop quality improvement approaches likely to have the greatest impact in a rural context. As discussed in Chapter 2, the committee is encouraging rural communities to develop communitywide collaborative approaches to prioritizing and addressing both personal and population health issues. Communities that pursue this approach may find it preferable to establish communitywide quality measurement and improvement programs, rather than having each provider setting develop its own approach. Communitywide quality programs may also have certain advantages in terms of the sharing or pooling of expertise and data.

To this end, the Department of Health and Human Services needs to develop a coordinated and tailored approach to meeting the needs of rural communities. Steps should also be taken to ensure that rural areas receive their fair share of quality improvement resources and technical assistance.

> **Recommendation 2. The Department of Health and Human Services should establish a Rural Quality Initiative to coordinate and accelerate efforts to measure and improve the quality of personal and population health care programs in rural areas. This initiative should be coordinated by the Health Resources and Services Administration's Office of Rural Health Policy, with guidance from a Rural Quality Advisory Panel consisting of experts from the private sector and state**

and local governments having knowledge and experience in rural health care quality measurement and improvement.

The agenda of this proposed initiative should include the following:

- *Application of evidence to practice*—AHRQ should assume a lead role in adapting clinical practice guidelines developed by professional associations and others to reflect the unique configuration of services, resource constraints, and challenges of rural areas, and in developing educational programs and tools to assist rural communities in applying evidence to practice.
- *Standardized measure set for rural communities*—The Rural Quality Advisory Panel should work collaboratively with public and private stakeholders (e.g., CMS, the Quality Interagency Coordinating Committee, AHRQ, the National Quality Forum, JCAHO, the National Committee for Quality Assurance) on the identification of appropriate standardized measures for rural areas, including (1) a subset of measures from leading measure sets that are applicable to rural areas; (2) where necessary, new rural-specific measures; and (3) standardized population health measures to be piloted in rural areas.
- *Public reporting*—CMS and the Rural Quality Advisory Panel should work collaboratively to ensure that rural providers are included in public reporting initiatives and that public reports for rural providers make fair and meaningful comparisons.
- *Community-based technical assistance*—CMS should ensure that the QIOs devote resources to rural areas commensurate with the proportion of Medicare beneficiaries in a state that reside in rural areas. Consideration should be given to establishing a QIOSC to focus on application of the above standardized rural quality measures to rural areas. The Office of Rural Health Policy should convene a series of regional conferences for critical access hospitals, rural health clinics, community health centers, and other providers to share quality improvement processes and techniques.
- *Data repository*—CMS should expand its data repositories to include rural-specific quality data so that rural providers have access to both urban and rural data for benchmarking purposes.

REFERENCES

AHQA (American Health Quality Association). 2004 (April 22). *AHQA Matters* (newsletter) 5(9). Washington, DC: American Health Quality Association.

AHRQ (Agency for Healthcare Research and Quality). 2003a. *National Healthcare Disparities Report*. [Online]. Available: http://qualitytools.ahrq.gov/disparities report/download_report.aspx [accessed July 7, 2004].

AHRQ. 2003b. *National Healthcare Quality Report*. Washington, DC: U.S. Department of Health and Human Services.

Brasure M, Stensland J, Wellever A. 2000. Quality oversight: Why are rural hospitals less likely to be JCAHO accredited? *Journal of Rural Health* 16(4):324–336.

Casey M, Moscovice I. 2004. *Quality Improvement Strategies and Best Practices in Critical Access Hospitals*. Minneapolis, MN: Rural Health Research Center, University of Minneapolis.

Chin MH, Cook S, Drum ML, Jin L, Guillen M, Humikowski CA, Koppert J, Harrison JF, Lippold S, Schaefer CT. 2004. Improving diabetes care in midwest community health centers with the health disparities collaborative. *Diabetes Care* 27(1):2–8.

CMS (Centers for Medicare and Medicaid Services). 2003a. *Reduce Disparities for Underserved and Rural Beneficiaries Project Description*. [Online]. Available: http://www.medqic.org/content/nationalpriorities/topics/projectdes.jsp?topicID=491&pageFrom=measures&pageID=3 [accessed May 14, 2004].

CMS. 2003b. *Quality Improvement Organizations: 6th Scope of Work*. [Online]. Available: http://www.cms.hhs.gov/qio/2a.pdf [accessed May 14, 2004].

CMS. 2004a. *Medicare Compare Databases*. [Online]. Available: http://www.medicare.gov/Download/DownloadDB.asp [accessed November 3, 2004].

CMS. 2004b. *Medicare Modernization Update: Medicare Prescription Drug, Improvement, and Modernization Act of 2003*. [Online]. Available: http://www.cms.hhs.gov/mmu/default.asp [accessed July 7, 2004].

Detmer DE, Singleton PD, Macleod A, Wait S, Taylor M, Ridwell J. 2003 (March). *The Informed Patient: Study Report*. Cambridge, UK: Judge Institute of Management, Cambridge University Health.

Federal Register. 2002. *Medicare and Medicaid Programs: Application by the Joint Commission on Accreditation of Healthcare Organizations for Approval of Deeming Authority for Critical Access Hospitals*. [Online]. Available: http://www.cms.hhs.gov/providerupdate/regs/cms2140pn.pdf [accessed July 7, 2004].

FMT (Flex Monitoring Team). 2004. *CAH Information: Complete List of Critical Access Hospitals*. [Online]. Available: http://flexmonitoring.org/cahlist [accessed July 7, 2004].

IOM (Institute of Medicine). 2003. *Health Professions Education: A Bridge to Quality*. Washington, DC: The National Academies Press.

JCAHO (Joint Commission on the Accreditation of Healthcare Organizations). 2004 (January). *Special Report: Shared Visions—New Pathways*. [Online]. Available: http://www.jcaho.org/accredited+organizations/svnp/jcp-2004-january.pdf [accessed January 2004].

Knott A, Travers K. 2002. *Implementing Quality Assessment and Performance Improvement Systems in Rural Health Clinics: Clinic and State Agency Responses*. Minneapolis, MN: Rural Health Research Center, University of Minnesota.

MedPAC (Medicare Payment Advisory Commission). 2001. *Report to the Congress: Medicare in Rural America*. Washington, DC: MedPAC.

Moscovice I, Casey M, Krein S. 1997. *Rural Managed Care: Patterns and Prospects*. Minneapolis, MN: Rural Health Research Center, University of Minnesota.

Moscovice I, Gregg WR, Klinger JM. 2002. *Rural Hospital Flexibility Program Tracking Project Year Three Report.* Chapter 3B: The Maturation of CAH Quality Assurance and Quality Improvement Strategies. Rural Policy Research Institute. Seattle, WA: WWAMI Rural Health Research Center, University of Washington.

Moscovice I, Wholey DR, Klingner J, Knott A. 2004. *Measuring Rural Hospital Quality.* Minneapolis, MN: Rural Health Research Center, University of Minnesota.

NACRHHS (National Advisory Committee on Rural Health and Human Services). 2001. *Medicare Reform: A Rural Perspective.* Washington, DC: Health Resources and Services Administration, U.S. Department of Health and Human Services.

NACRHHS. 2003. *Health Care Quality: The Rural Context.* Washington, DC: Health Resources and Services Administration, U.S. Department of Health and Human Services.

NQF (National Quality Forum). 2003. *Safe Practices for Better Healthcare: A Consensus Report.* Washington, DC: NQF.

Stratis Health. 2004. *2003–2004 Critical Access Hospital Collaborative.* [Online]. Available: http://www.stratishealth.org/health-care/documents/CAHCollaborative_FinalReport_June2004_000.pdf [accessed July 7, 2004].

USDHHS (U.S. Department of Health and Human Services). 2001. *Health, United States 2001 with Urban and Rural Health Chartbook.* Washington, DC: U.S. Government Printing Office.

4

Human Resources

SUMMARY

An adequate supply of properly educated health care professionals is critical to meeting the health needs of rural and frontier communities. Experientially based education programs should be enhanced to ensure that all health professionals master the core competencies necessary to provide high-quality care (i.e., provide patient-centered care, work in interdisciplinary teams, employ evidence-based practice, apply quality improvement, and utilize informatics).

Efforts should also be made to boost the supply of health professionals in rural areas. A multifaceted approach to the recruitment and retention of health professionals is needed, including interventions at every point along the rural workforce pipeline: (1) enhanced preparation of rural elementary and high school students to pursue health careers; (2) stronger commitment of health professions education programs to recruiting students from rural areas, educating and training students in rural areas, and adopting rural-appropriate curricula; and (3) stronger incentives for health professionals to seek and retain employment in rural areas.

Lastly, steps should be taken to build stronger rural health communities that mobilize all types of human resources (e.g., patients and family caregivers) and institutions (e.g., educational, social, and faith-based) to both augment and support the contributions of health professionals.

Human resources are critical to every rural community's efforts to improve individual and population health. Human resources include health care professionals, both those in practice and those in training, as well as the population at large in the community.

The recruitment and retention of an adequate supply of properly trained health care professionals are essential for the delivery of quality health care. Although advances in information and communications technology (ICT) hold promise for providing rural residents with remote access to many specialists and services (see Chapter 6), a good deal of health care is best provided locally. The provision of many essential health care services—preventive and primary care, surgical and hospital care, chronic care management, and emergency care—relies to varying degrees on the availability of health care professionals with the appropriate education and skills to provide care competently.

For decades, rural and frontier communities have struggled to attract and retain an adequate supply of the various health care professionals that make up the rural health care team, including family physicians, nurse professionals, physician assistants, emergency care specialists, mental and behavioral health professionals, pharmacists, and dentists. (Appendix C provides detailed information on the availability of various types of health professionals in rural areas.) Some success has been achieved in attracting certain types of health care professionals, while shortages of others have grown worse. Demographic trends make it essential that greater efforts be made to address the health professional workforce needs of rural communities. Many rural communities are experiencing an increase in residents over age 65 as a result of the aging of the population and in-migration of retirees from the "baby boom" generation (see Appendix B). Unless steps are taken soon, there will likely be a widening gap between the available numbers of health care providers and the numbers required to meet the needs of rural populations. The aging of the population and the associated increase in persons with multiple chronic conditions also make it imperative that steps be taken soon to establish better methods of communication and information sharing among the providers in a community.

There is no doubt that the health care professional workforce is important, but so, too, is the broader set of human resources in rural communities. As discussed in Chapter 2, to achieve significant improvements in health, rural communities will need to pursue initiatives aimed at improving both population health and the quality of the personal health care system. Rural residents and other community stakeholders (e.g., social service agencies, educational institutions, faith-based organizations) play a pivotal role at each of these levels in determining health care needs and outcomes. Of particular importance are the health-related knowledge and skills of a rural community's population and the tools and supports available to individuals to manage their health needs.

This chapter includes four sections. The first provides an overview of fundamental reforms in health professions education and training needed to improve quality of care and explains their particular relevance to rural communities. The second provides an overview of the points along the rural workforce pipeline and identifies a set of interventions that should be pursued to increase the supply and enhance the skill set of rural health professionals. The third describes various options for mobilizing a broader set of human resources—those of the population at large and those resident within other social institutions (e.g., social service agencies, educational institutions, faith-based organizations)—to improve health and health care in rural communities. The final section presents conclusions and recommendations.

FUNDAMENTAL REFORMS TO IMPROVE QUALITY

Fundamental changes within health professions education are needed to better prepare clinicians to respond to the population's needs and address shortcomings in quality—changes that are important to both urban and rural communities. The focus of the health care needs of the American population has been shifting for several decades from acute illnesses to chronic conditions. The management of chronic conditions calls for a model of health care delivery that (1) actively engages patients and family caregivers and offers them educational, psychosocial, and other supports for the ongoing management of these conditions, and (2) provides coordinated care through multidisciplinary teams.

In addition to the changing needs of the population, there has been an exponential increase in the science base that supports health care (IOM, 2001). Many of today's quality shortcomings stem from a failure to provide clinicians with the educational and organizational supports required to remain current with the evidence base and apply the evidence appropriately to practice (DiCenso et al., 1998; Evers, 2001; Haynes, 2002; Jadad and Haynes, 1998; Lang, 1999; Mazurek, 2002). The *Quality Chasm* report (IOM, 2001) asserts that achieving the highest quality of care possible is predicated on both the redesign of systems of care and a workforce that is fully prepared to function in these new systems (IOM, 2001). To function in redesigned rural health care systems that consistently deliver quality care, health professionals will need to have knowledge and skills that have not historically been part of health professions and health management education, but are essential to moving the quality agenda forward in both rural health care environments and rural communities.

Core Competencies for Health Professionals

In 2002, the IOM convened a summit of leaders from the health professions, primarily medicine, nursing, allied health, and pharmacy, to identify changes in health professions education and training required to achieve the vision of high-quality care set forth in the *Quality Chasm* report. Participants at the summit identified five core competencies that all health professionals should possess (see Box 4-1). Educational programs at all levels (i.e., undergraduate, graduate, and continuing education) should focus greater attention on these core competencies. Although these competencies are relevant for clinicians in all geographic areas, the way they are operationalized by providers may be influenced by the characteristics of the practice setting, including rural versus urban. Substantial work will be required to ensure the consistent acquisition and application of these competencies across rural settings.

BOX 4-1
Core Competencies for
Health Professionals

- Provide patient-centered care
- Work in interdisciplinary teams
- Employ evidence-based practice
- Apply quality improvement
- Utilize informatics

SOURCE: IOM, 2003c.

Provide Patient-Centered Care

This competency requires knowing and respecting patients' differences, values, preferences, and expressed needs. The focus is on shared decision making and care management. Research indicates that patients involved in care decisions and management have better health outcomes, lower costs, and higher functional status than those not thus involved (Bodenheimer et al., 2002a,b; Lorig et al., 1999). This competency also incorporates a focus on population health.

To provide patient-centered care, clinicians must have cultural competency and familiarity with key facets of the lives and environments of rural residents. Because familiarity with many members of the community is common in rural areas, clinicians, from office nurses to pharmacists, are often knowledgeable about patients' social, cultural, and family characteristics. Recent studies confirm a sizable proportion of minority patients report problems in communicating with clinicians of different ethnic and racial backgrounds, and as a result, do not fully understand the physician's written instructions or follow medical advice (Collins et al., 2002; Cooper et al., 2003; IOM, 2003a). Similar problems likely arise when the "cultural divide" is one related to rural versus urban background. As discussed later in this chapter, many steps can and should be taken to enable and encourage rural residents to pursue health professions careers, and this is one strategy to enhance patient-centered care. However, for the foreseeable future, it is likely that rural health systems will rely on clinicians with many different cultural backgrounds, and from urban areas and foreign countries. This makes it particularly important that education and training programs, especially experiential, rural community-based programs, place sufficient emphasis on enhancing the cultural competency and communication skills of all providers.

This competency is closely linked to one of the ten simple rules for the twenty-first century health care system set forth in the *Quality Chasm* report. This rule identifies the patient as the source of control, with care being customized based on patient needs and values. Since there is a lower proportion of individuals with formal education in rural communities (see Appendix B), patients and families may need more guidance and support to ensure understanding of their choices as they make decisions about their care and to maximize their ability to engage in self-management.

Given the fairly well-defined composition of rural communities served by local health care clinicians, rural health care systems may be well positioned to take a population focus, including engaging the local community in determining its needs and preferences for health care services. Knowledge of what drives rural residents' utilization of services, of community risk factors, and of health status and other population characteristics can inform customized illness prevention and health promotion efforts at the community level, as well as appropriate behavioral changes.

Work in Interdisciplinary Teams

This competency involves health professionals from varied disciplines who collaborate, communicate, and integrate care to ensure consistent, high quality. An interdisciplinary approach is especially relevant to rural health care given the higher frequency of chronic illness in rural versus urban populations (USAC, 2004). The involvement of a range of clinicians with varying knowledge, skills, and experience is particularly important to the ongoing management of patients with chronic conditions. In addition to care for chronic illness, an interdisciplinary team approach is important for the provision of acute care, such as when a patient in the immediate care of rural emergency medical technicians is transported to the emergency room of a rural or urban hospital. Acquiring this competency is also important for rural clinicians given that team approaches have been linked to key quality improvements, including greater concordance with complex treatment protocols for the chronically ill, decreased risk-adjusted lengths of stay in intensive care units, and impact on patient safety and reduction of medical errors (IOM, 2003c).

One distinctive feature of many rural health care settings is the broader scope of practice for primary care providers and the greater use of midlevel professionals (e.g., nurse practitioners) and technicians (e.g., pharmacy and physical therapy technicians) (see Appendix C). In the area of mental health, for example, primary care physicians provide the majority of services (Hartley et al., 1999). When such services are provided by mental health professionals, rural areas often rely on social workers and psychiatric nurses, whereas urban areas tend to have a greater complement of psychiatrists and psychologists.

In redesigned health systems, rural teams must have effective methods of providing supervision, expert consultation, and emergency backup to offer patients seamless care regardless of the setting or team member engaged with the patient at any given time. All team members must have strong communication skills and a clear understanding of each other's roles and responsibilities. In rural settings, it is not uncommon for health care workers to know each other and to have worked together for years, a situation intensified by the markedly smaller number of clinicians and managers involved. Yet competency in team care requires much more than familiarity. It involves learning approaches to maximize collaborative work; ensuring that timely information reaches those who need it; and managing patient transitions across settings and over time, even when team members are in different physical locations. Because rural health care services frequently are based in a single organization—typically the local hospital—that provides an array of services from home health to outpatient to nursing home care, rural team members in many settings often have easier access to one another and closer communication as patients move across care sectors. When specialty or subspecialty care is involved, however, it is not uncommon for clinicians to be communicating with other providers located 50 or 100 miles away. Ensuring that all relevant information from the distant site accompanies the patient back to the rural community can be problematic, and open communication can be inhibited. Ensuring that team concepts and processes are employed under these circumstances may be more challenging.

Employ Evidence-Based Practice

Providing evidence-based care requires that clinicians be skilled in accessing the current knowledge base, including literature syntheses (e.g., Cochrane Collaboratives) and practice guidelines promulgated by professional organizations and other reputable sources (French, 1999; Grad et al., 2001; Rosswurm and Larrabee, 1999; Walshe and Rundall, 2001). This competency further requires that clinicians be able to integrate evidence with clinical expertise and patient values.

As the science base has grown and the complexity of care has increased, it is apparent that applying science appropriately to practice for every patient requires carefully designed care processes. Indeed, this competency relates directly to another of the ten simple rules alluded to above: that decision making is evidence-based, with clinicians providing care and administrators facilitating system redesign on the basis of scientific knowledge.

Prerequisite to this competency is having access to current evidence. Historically, this competency has been difficult to achieve for clinicians in many rural environments because of a lack of such access. Because they are often few in number, clinicians in rural areas can have difficulty obtaining coverage to attend regional or national educational conferences. Likewise, rural facilities have traditionally been beyond the scope of educational opportunities such as grand rounds and in-house presentations that are common to teaching hospitals and other entities.

The availability of the Internet and web-based information from such sources as the Agency for Healthcare Research and Quality now gives the rural workforce virtually the same opportunities as their urban counterparts to access the latest information and ensure that their patients will receive services based on the most current evidence available. However, the application of some research to rural patients and settings can be problematic. Much of the quality research on clinical care and health care management, for example, has been done in tertiary care settings and may not reflect the structures and processes common to rural health care delivery. Furthermore, the application of evidence to practice in rural settings can be challenging given the time constraints of clinicians, the lack of clinical librarians, and the part-time status of some clinicians. Additionally, because of the low volume of patients seen in many rural facilities, it is not uncommon to find clinicians who must maintain current knowledge across a range of practice areas. Caring for individuals with health problems that present far less frequently in rural settings also poses a special challenge to the members of the health care team, who must ensure that they maintain their knowledge and proficiency in the context of rural resources and the relative lack of organizational support.

Apply Quality Improvement

All health care professionals should possess a basic knowledge of quality improvement theory and the ability to employ quality measurement and improvement tools in their practice, including measuring quality in terms of structure, process, and outcomes in relation to patient and community needs. Improving patient safety (i.e., reducing errors), for example, involves (1) developing a culture of safety in the health care system that encourages and rewards individual and organizational behavior directed at safety improvements, (2) establishing reporting and analysis systems to capture near misses and injuries and to conduct root-cause analyses to identify the factors that contributed to errors, and (3) redesigning care processes to reduce the likelihood of errors occurring and mitigate harm when they do occur (IOM, 2004d).

This competency links to another of the ten simple rules: that safety is a system property whereby health professionals engage in system redesign efforts to prevent and mitigate errors and decrease resource waste. Rural areas have characteristics that make achieving this end different in some respects than in urban settings. In rural health settings, leadership in quality assurance and improvement efforts often rests with a senior clinician who is responsible for multiple tasks. This can represent a challenge given that quality improvement requires knowledge of the field, along with the ability to assess current practices and compare them with those of other providers and facilities, to design and implement process changes, and to incorporate

safety design principles such as human factors-related training and standardization.

In rural areas, information relevant to quality improvement may be ac-
cessed through networks of rural and/or urban facilities sharing such resources; through Quality Improvement Organizations (QIOs); or, in the case
of critical access hospitals, the use of federal funds available through the
Rural Hospital Flexibility Program. For example, sharing information across
a number of geographically dispersed facilities in Montana allows the pooling and application of expertise and acquired knowledge. Furthermore, physicians in some rural communities in states such as North Dakota engage in
peer review of the work of colleagues, not necessarily within their own facility, but in similar facilities across significant geographic distances. Increasingly, rural facilities are building such networks to pool limited resources
and maximize access to expertise for quality improvement purposes, further
demonstrating the high value of networking and collaboration among rural
health organizations and with urban facilities.

As mentioned earlier, the competency to apply quality improvement is
linked to decreasing the waste of resources, including money, time, and
ideas. While some may view rural health care facilities as efficient, even
with such circumstances as fixed overhead and low service volume, waste
can be identified in rural care processes. For example, when a patient is
stabilized and subsequently transferred from a rural hospital emergency
room to an urban hospital, it is not uncommon for laboratory and other
tests to be repeated at the urban facility. Likewise, to meet internal rules
and external requirements, multiple transfer forms are completed in many
rural facilities as part of the transfer process. The competency to apply quality improvement encompasses the ability to address both overuse of services and inefficient redundancies.

The focus of quality improvement and the processes by which it is implemented in rural facilities may differ from the urban case given the differences in organizational structure, processes, workforce, and patient mix.
Consequently, applying the quality improvement literature in rural environments may require additional steps on the part of rural providers to ensure
appropriateness, relevance, and success in implementation. One potential
advantage of the application of quality improvement in rural settings is that
while large facilities often adopt new practices on a unit-by-unit basis, the
size of rural facilities may allow system-wide adoption to be accomplished
more quickly and efficiently.

Finally, if the rural workforce is to deliver high-quality care, it must be led by individuals and boards who want and expect innovation, understand the essential ingredients in improving quality, and ensure that the workforce has the time and the resources to acquire the necessary knowledge and skills. Infrastructure support is essential as well to assist providers in accessing and incorporating an ever-expanding knowledge and technology base.

Utilize Informatics

Building an ICT infrastructure to support care delivery is critical to achieving the six quality aims (see Chapter 6). ICT also links to another of the ten simple rules—that knowledge is shared and information flows freely. Elements of an ICT infrastructure for health care include electronic health records, clinical decision-support tools, and telehealth capabilities, with a focus on such areas as knowledge management, error reduction, and information acquisition. Such an ICT infrastructure has far-reaching implications for the way in which care is delivered and for the roles of health professionals and patients.

With some exceptions, rural health care continues to be dominated by paper-based information. Yet given the established links that generally exist across a small set of health care providers within rural communities, there is great potential to automate those links and enable information to be readily shared. Health care professionals must appreciate the importance of ICT to delivering high-quality care and have the knowledge and skills to acquire ICT and use it effectively in their practices. This is particularly important in rural areas, where the typical practice setting is very small, and access to technical expertise in ICT is limited. Moreover, clinicians' access to technology such as telemedicine and email can be challenging in communities that have limited infrastructure linking them to high-speed lines. These structural issues can limit access to services in rural communities that do not have the personnel to staff critical care units, radiologists available around the clock, or mental health care providers such as psychiatrists available in the immediate community.

Programs to Provide the Core Competencies

The five core competencies are relevant to health care professionals at all stages of their career—as students, recent graduates, and seasoned clinicians—and to a great extent are acquired through experiential learning programs. Such programs will need to be established at the community level and engage all providers in the community. Rural communities offer excellent opportunities to establish such programs for several reasons. First, they are generally less complex than urban environments because of their smaller size and scale. Second, the scarcity of providers in rural communities should facilitate collaboration. Third, as discussed in Chapter 3, in rural areas many quality measurement and improvement activities need to involve the entire community because individual practice settings have insufficient sample sizes and expertise to support those activities. The development of such experiential learning programs should proceed in tandem with the establishment of an ICT infrastructure (see Chapter 6).

The Health Resources and Services Administration (HRSA) administers dozens of grant programs to increase the supply and enhance the training of health professionals, especially those willing to work in areas designated as having too few providers, as well as those who are members of an ethnic or racial minority group or who come from a disadvantaged background. Most but not all of these programs are authorized under Titles VII and VIII of the Public Health Service Act, and they are funded at a relatively modest level (approximately $289.5 million in fiscal year 2004) (BHPR, 2004d,e; HRSA, 2004a,b,c). Few target rural communities directly, so it is unclear the extent to which rural communities benefit. Several federal grant programs provide modest financial support for interdisciplinary training in rural communities. In the past decade, the Quentin Burdick Rural Program for Interdisciplinary Training has trained about 13,000 practicing clinicians, teachers, and students in 29 states through demonstration programs, with area health education centers often being the grantees in collaboration with other community-based organizations (BHPR, 2004d). In fiscal year 2003, the program awarded 23 grants for a total of $6.2 million. There are also a number of federal grant programs that support interdisciplinary training at specific sites, including HRSA's Area Health Education Centers (often located in medical schools), Health Education and Training Centers in the southwestern border region ($4 million for 13 projects in fiscal year 2003), and Geriatric Education Centers ($15.6 million for 46 projects in fiscal year 2003) (BHPR, 2004a,b,c). A number of states also support interdisciplinary training programs (Buckwalter, 2004).

These programs, especially the Quentin Burdick Rural Program for Interdisciplinary Training, provide a foundation upon which to build. Additional support will be required to accomplish the objective of providing experiential training in the five core competencies for all clinicians in rural areas.

Additionally, organizations that focus on health care for rural communities, such as the National Rural Health Association, the small and rural hospitals section of the American Hospital Association, the State Offices of Rural Health, and the federally funded Rural Assistance Center (http://www.raconline.org) could serve as information conduits to help providers acquire the core competencies. Organizations with a quality focus, such as the Institute for Safe Medication Practices, the Institute for Healthcare Improvement, the Agency for Healthcare Research and Quality, and others, could target efforts to rural audiences. As discussed in Chapter 3, QIOs might provide greater technical assistance to rural providers in acquiring quality improvement knowledge and techniques. Lastly, it is important to recognize that educational supports can be provided through distance learning programs. Internet-based educational opportunities for health professionals have expanded greatly in recent years, as has the technology for interactive distance learning. The committee does not view distance education programs as a substitute for community-based experiential training programs, but does think distance education should be explored as a way to help health professionals retain and build upon the core competencies initially acquired through the latter programs (although it should be noted that some state licensure programs limit the use of distance education in satisfying continuing medical education requirements [AMA, 2002]). The committee recognizes that there are advantages and disadvantages to distance learning, but does encourage states and other regulatory bodies to periodically re-evaluate this option as distance education programs and technologies evolve.

ENHANCING THE RURAL HEALTH PROFESSIONS WORKFORCE

The model for achieving greater numbers of rural clinicians is often conceptualized in terms of a pipeline, with each point along the pipeline playing an essential part in achieving the ultimate goal of increasing the size of the rural workforce and its capacity to provide high-quality health care (see Figure 4-1). The points shown in Figure 4-1 can be aggregated into three broad areas: (1) attracting rural students to health careers, (2) providing formal education programs, and (3) recruiting and retraining trained health professionals in rural areas. The IOM committee believes there are opportunities to make improvements in each of these links that will enhance the supply of health professionals in rural areas and to improve their competency in the five core areas discussed above.

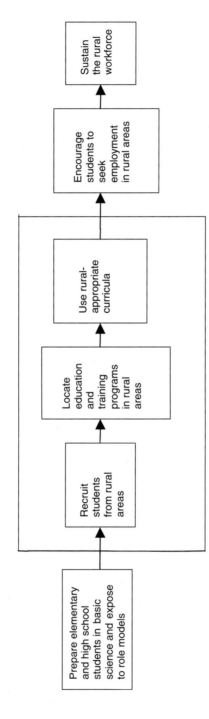

FIGURE 4-1 The rural workforce pipeline.
SOURCE: Hart et al., 2002.

Measures to Attract Rural Students to Health Careers

There is evidence to indicate that people from rural communities who become health professionals are more likely to choose to practice in rural areas after completing their formal education and to remain in rural practice for longer periods of time then their nonrural counterparts (Rabinowtiz et al., 2001). Measures to attract rural students to health careers involve enrichment of schooling for precollegiate students, ensuring that basic science is part of the curriculum and that students have positive exposure to role models and career paths in rural health care delivery. For students who choose not to enroll in health professions training, such exposure contributes to increased health literacy and lays the groundwork for local residents to become more engaged and informed participants in health promotion and health care delivery in their communities.

Over the last two decades, a great deal of attention has been focused on enhancing science education in grades K through 12 (Hart et al., 2003; NRC, 1996, 2002, 2003). In 1996, the Department of Education promulgated National Science Education Standards to serve as guidelines for states and local districts in developing their own, more specific standards, curriculum, and implementation processes. Many of the nation's schools are enhancing their science curricula. Responses to a 2000 survey indicated that 46 states had developed new science content standards, but only 4 states required 4 science credits for graduation (compared with 18 states that required 2 credits and 16 that required 1.5–3.5 credits) (NRC, 2003). By the time of graduation, 95 percent of students had completed a biology course, 54 percent in chemistry (versus 45 percent in 1990) and 23 percent in physics (versus 20 percent in 1990). Enrollment of African Americans and Hispanics in higher-level classes continued to lag behind that of Caucasians and Asians across the board. Results specific to rural and urban areas are not available.

There are a handful of innovative programs that expose elementary and high school students from rural areas to health professions information and role models. These include programs that provide volunteer ambulance corps assignments for high school and elementary students from rural areas (New York); send teams of health professions students to teach health education and discuss careers with rural adolescents at 4-H summer camps (Tennessee); enroll minority and lower-income high school students in the Health Sciences and Technology Academy; and provide summer health careers education through local science clubs (West Virginia) (Gamm et al., 2002). The Academy also supports science teachers by helping them learn better teaching skills to maintain their students' interest in science and math. Formal evaluation of these programs is needed to assess their success in recruiting rural students into the health professions.

Formal Education Programs

The supply of health care professionals is influenced by both the capacity of health professions education programs and the structure and content of these programs. Studies of the geographic distribution of health professionals confirm that as their overall supply increases, so, too, does the diffusion of clinicians into rural areas. For example, early studies of physician diffusion found that as the supply of physicians grew during the 1970s, many chose to practice in rural areas, so that by 1979, nearly every small town (with a population of more than 2,500) had ready access to a physician (Newhouse et al., 1982). This finding has been corroborated by recent studies showing that as the supply of physicians doubled between 1979 and 1999, geographic access continued to improve (Rosenthal et al., 2003).

It is important to note, however, that the relationship between increased supply and greater geographic distribution is, to a great extent, specialty specific. That is, as the supply of physicians of a particular specialty increases, physicians of that specialty are more likely to seek practice in rural areas. This is an important caveat for rural areas. As discussed above, rural areas rely to a great extent on family physicians, and this is the one specialty that experienced a steady and progressive decline in numbers from 1980 through 1999 (Biola et al., 2003).

The structure and content of health professions education programs also influence a clinician's likelihood of choosing rural practice and preparedness to provide high-quality care in rural settings. First, as noted above, recruitment of qualified students from rural communities influences the choice of practice setting. Second, the likelihood of health professionals choosing to practice in rural areas is also increased if they are able to remain in rural areas while obtaining some or all of their professional education (Hart et al., 2002). Third, to adequately prepare health professionals to practice in rural areas, education programs must recruit faculty with rural practice experience and develop appropriate curricula.

An important aspect of preparing and recruiting future health professionals from rural communities is creating opportunities for members of minority and disadvantaged populations, such as American Indians, Alaska Natives, and African, Hispanic, and Asian Americans, who may be overrepresented in rural versus urban locales and underrepresented among rural providers. As noted earlier, HRSA administers a number of programs aimed at recruiting students from such backgrounds. These include loan repayment and scholarship programs, as well as grant programs that support recruitment and training of such students and future faculty at schools and affiliated training programs (BHPR, 2004b). Additionally, the Indian Health Service (IHS) offers a range of programs across the spectrum of health professions, encompassing undergraduate preparatory training, externships, and health professions scholarship and loan repayment, to students who are members of federally recognized tribes, and gives hiring preference to tribe members (BHPR, 2004b).

These programs can be further augmented with improvement in the policies and practices that govern the admissions processes of health professions educational programs as recommended in the 2004 IOM report, *In the Nation's Compelling Interest: Ensuring Diversity in the Health Care Workforce*. This earlier IOM report recommends that:

> Admissions should be based on a comprehensive review of each applicant. Such attributes include, but are not limited to, applicants' race or ethnicity, socioeconomic background, cross-cultural experience, life choices, multilingual abilities, interpersonal skills, cultural competence, leadership qualities, barriers the applicant has overcome, and other attributes that reflect the institutional mission. Admissions models should balance quantitative data (i.e., prior grades and standardized test scores) with these qualitative characteristics (IOM, 2004c, p. 85).

Health professions educational programs are encouraged to examine their admissions practices to ensure that the criteria for admission are well balanced and consistent with the program's overall objectives. In addition, additional study should be undertaken to better understand the relative contribution of various types of factors, both quantitative and qualitative, in identifying prospective candidates likely to complete the educational program successfully and to pursue careers in rural areas.

Following is a brief discussion of current formal education programs for generalist physicians, nurses, physician assistants, emergency care professionals, dentists, pharmacists, mental and behavioral health care professionals, health administrators, and public health professionals as they pertain to building the rural health care workforce.

Physicians

For physicians, two factors are strongly predictive of a future career in rural health: a rural background and plans to enter family medicine

(Rabinowitz and Taylor, 2004). With regard to medical school training, other important predictive factors include the commitment of the medical school to rural practice (public schools in rural states are more likely to have such a commitment than are private research schools in urban areas), provision of training in family medicine, experienced faculty role models or mentors with a rural focus, required rural experiential learning at different stages of training, and the presence of advisors to assist with the transition to a rural residency (Hart et al., 2002; Hartley et al., 1999; WHA, 2004).

Medical schools that make a strong commitment to educating physicians for rural practice have quite successful track records. Jefferson Medical College's Physician Shortage Area Program (PSAP) in Philadelphia, which recruits and provides financial assistance to rural students and offers focused training in family medicine (mentoring, rural clerkships, and preceptorships), produces graduates that are more than 8.5 times as likely to work in rural family medicine than Jefferson's non-PSAP graduates (Liederman and Morefield, 2003; Rabinowitz and Taylor, 2004). Other examples include the Rural Physician Program (Michigan State University), which places 8 students annually at clinical training sites in the Upper Peninsula; the Rural Medical Education Program (University of Illinois College of Medicine at Rockford), which admits up to 15 students each year for training that includes early and sustained participation in ambulatory primary care at rural sites and rural preceptorships; the University of North Dakota, which places 7 students in the third year of medical school in a 7-month rural experience known as ROME (Rural Opportunities in Medical Education); and the Rural/Underserved Opportunities program, which offers clinical placement and clerkships at rural sites in Spokane, Washington, and Boise, Idaho (WHA, 2004). It may be noted that osteopaths are overrepresented among all physicians in rural areas, reflecting the orientation of their training toward primary care of underserved groups and rural clinical sites for training (Tooke-Rawlins, 2000).

The factors noted above as predictive of a future career in rural health are not the norm in residency and other postgraduate training. Most residency training takes place in urban teaching hospitals, and the majority of public (federal and state) financing of residency training through Medicare and Medicaid graduate medical education (GME) programs flows to hospitals in urban settings. In 1998, only about 3 percent of acute care hospitals in nonmetropolitan counties (70 hospitals) participated in Medicare GME, compared with almost 40 percent of hospitals in metropolitan areas (NRHA, 2003). The committee concurs with others that the nearly $14 billion in public funds spent annually ($6 billion through Medicare, $4 billion through Medicaid, plus more than $4 billion in state support to allopathic medical schools) to educate 22,000 physicians could be better targeted to achieve rural workforce goals (Myers, 2000; NRHA, 2003).

An earlier IOM committee examined alternatives for better aligning public financing of GME with the attainment of health care workforce goals (IOM, 2004a). Two options were considered:

• *Incremental change in existing payment programs*—For example, the Medicare program's direct and indirect GME programs could be tied more closely to the training of family physicians (who are more likely to practice in rural settings) or to the training of residents in rural hospitals. This approach maintains a link with an entitlement program (i.e., "automatic" funding), but has the disadvantage of trying to achieve workforce goals through a payment program established with other objectives in mind.

• *Fundamental change*—For example, health workforce subsidization might be removed from the Medicare payment program and replaced with a separate program designed specifically to achieve public policy goals. In theory, this approach would allow for the setting of national workforce goals and the structuring of a financing program to meet those goals, while one of the major disadvantages is that medical education would have to compete with other budget priorities in the appropriations process.

The earlier IOM committee concluded that it is unlikely that an entirely new funding source would be created and that the best course would be to pursue incremental change in existing payment programs. This committee concurs and, specifically, encourages Congress and the administration to be particularly attentive to the needs of rural communities when pursuing incremental reform.

In addition to a commitment to training more generalists for rural practice, there must be a commitment to meeting the needs of rural populations for specialty care. To some extent, specialty needs can be met through cross-training of generalists. For example, family physicians and general surgeons can receive subspecialty training in emergency medicine (Williams et al., 2001). Likewise, pediatricians can be cross-trained to provide dental services, as is the case in one West Virginia community (Fos and Hutchison, 2003; Gordon, 2004). The numbers of certain types of specialists, such as psychiatrists, might be increased by establishing residency programs for those specialties with rotations in rural settings (Hartley et al., 1999). The creation of networks linking specialist physicians serving rural areas with those in urban settings is also an important element of building the health infrastructure in a way that can better support both physicians and patients.

Nurses

The rubric of nursing encompasses a variety of health professionals, from nursing assistants and licensed practical nurses with less than an associate's degree, to registered nurses with associate's and bachelor's degrees, to advanced practice nurses with master's- or doctoral-level training and state or national certification (such as clinical nurse specialists, practitioners, certified nurse midwives, and certified registered nurse anesthetists) (IOM, 2003d). For these professionals, as for physicians, characteristics associated with success in rural practice include a rural background or upbringing and health professions training in a rural environment (Hart et al., 2002).

An example of an innovative program for training nurse professionals is the University of Iowa's Registered Nurse-Bachelor of Science in Nursing Satellite Program, which trains rural students in their community of residence rather than requiring that they relocate to urban areas for schooling (Buckwalter, 2004). This program involves partnerships with community colleges, private health care agencies in Iowa and nearby states, and the University of Iowa's Colleges of Nursing and Pharmacy, and uses distance learning and mentoring faculty.

Physician Assistants

Compared with nurse practitioners, physician assistants are trained in a more diverse range of settings, from medical schools and schools of allied health to community colleges and the military (Hooker, 2002). Federal (Title VII) and many state scholarship and loan forgiveness programs serve as incentives to recruit physician assistants to rural communities (see the section below on recruitment and retention). Yet while a greater proportion of physician assistants practice in rural areas relative to the proportion of the total physician population, there is a trend toward choosing urban practice locations among physician assistants (Baer and Smith, 1999). In recent years, two innovative training programs for physician assistants have added rural curricula and place-based, experiential training through the use of web-based distance education and local clinical mentors:

- Since 1994, the Partnerships for Training Program, sponsored by The Robert Wood Johnson Foundation, has supported web-based distance education and clinical preceptorships based at satellite campuses in underserved areas (rural and urban) for physician assistant students (Johnson, 2002). As of 2002, 450 students had graduated, with at least 70 percent practicing in their communities.

- In the late 1990s, the College of Health Sciences in Roanoke, Virginia, which graduates many of the baccalaureate-level health providers in the region (rural central Appalachia), added a community focus and web-based management of student clinical participation to its new physician assistant training program (Dezendorf and Scott, 2001). During their second year of training, students participate in month-long community health clinical rotations in two small Virginia towns, completing distance coursework during nights and weekends, and spending 2 days per week of clinical activity supervised by a physician with rural expertise and 3 days per week directly participating in a community health project. The program features web-based updates on work progress and communication with other students, faculty, and community residents.

Emergency Care Professionals

There are two groups of emergency medical services (EMS) providers: prehospital providers and hospital-based teams. Prehospital EMS providers include first responders, ambulance attendants and drivers, and emergency care technicians with basic, intermediate, or paramedic training (Rural EMS Initiative, 2000). The level of certification of EMS providers in rural areas varies considerably, such that a responding team in one area may have only basic emergency medical technicians (EMTs) available, while that in another area may include a paramedic, regardless of the health needs of the patient. In rural areas, many prehospital EMS providers are volunteers. Recent years have seen some efforts to make formal EMS training more accessible to rural providers. To address rural concerns that the typical 2-year length of training for paramedics discourages local enrollees from seeking advanced training, the State of California has implemented modular or discrete instructional units that are flexible to accommodate the schedules of volunteers (Franks et al., 2004). ICT-based distance learning has been demonstrated to be comparable to on-site classroom training and can be used for either initial training or continuing education, with the advantage of keeping EMS staff in the field (Franks et al., 2004). Such training also enhances the future rural labor pool, for many volunteer technicians use their EMS experience as a stepping stone to education and work in other health care careers or in hospital or clinic settings (Franks et al., 2004).

Staffing hospital-based EMS services is also challenging. The need for 24-hour availability and the low volume of patients make it difficult for rural hospitals to hire specialists in emergency medicine and muster the financial resources to adequately support an EMS system (Moorhead et al., 2002; Rawlinson and Crews, 2003).

Training more specialist physicians in emergency medicine oriented toward rural practice—through new residency programs and clinical training sites—may be less feasible than expanding the content of family medicine or primary care residencies to encompass cross-training in emergency care. This cross-training could include certification of subspecialty training (in advanced cardiac life support, advanced trauma life support, and advanced pediatric life support) and training in interdisciplinary collaboration with the nurse professionals and physician assistants who make up a sizable proportion of the EMS workforce (Williams et al., 2001).

There is also a need to train emergency medicine physicians in urban areas that are adjacent to rural areas to provide support and backup for all types of clinicians in rural areas who must deal with emergency care needs. As discussed in Chapter 6, ICT is opening up many opportunities for enhanced collaboration between rural and urban areas.

Dentists

Both IHS and HRSA offer a variety of scholarship and loan repayment programs targeting dentists and dental hygienists. These programs include support for postgraduate residencies and interdisciplinary training, as well as for training of ethnic and racial minority group members underrepresented in the workforce, although the support for these programs is relatively modest (NACRHHS, 2004). There are a number of innovative education programs aimed at increasing the supply of dentists and dental hygienists:

• Nebraska has created a Midwest consortium for dental student education and financing that recruits from rural areas of Nebraska, South Dakota, Kansas, and Wyoming (Gordon, 2004).
• The University of Colorado School of Dentistry includes a 6- to 18-week clinical rotation in a rural community both to provide rural residents

with access to care and to increase the likelihood that students will choose a rural practice location (Gordon, 2004).

- A program in West Virginia provides pediatricians and school nurses with cross-training in dental care so they can deliver oral health screening and treatment services (Fos and Hutchison, 2003; Gordon, 2004).

Pharmacists

After nurses and physicians, pharmacists are the third-largest group of health professionals (196,000 active in the United States in 2000) (Hart et al., 2002; HRSA, 2000; USDHHS, 2000). In recent years, the roles and expected functions of pharmacists have expanded as a result of many factors, including the increased complexity of drug prescribing and management due to the greater numbers of pharmacological agents, and concerns about medication safety, especially in light of the sizable numbers of people being treated with complex, multifaceted medication regimens. A longer period of training for pharmacists to earn a doctorate is now the norm, and postgraduate residencies are common (Cooksey et al., 2002). One survey of retail pharmacists in three rural states (Minnesota, North Dakota, and South Dakota) found that 95 percent had a bachelor's degree (Casey et al., 2001).

Meeting the pharmacy needs of rural areas through training will involve collaboration between schools of pharmacy and rural areas, given that, as with other health professions, students from rural areas are more likely to choose rural practice (Scott et al., 1992). The enhanced role of pharmacists beyond the simple dispensing of prescriptions requires not only new and different training than in the past, but also increased cross-training with other health care students to facilitate interdisciplinary team work, including telesupervision by pharmacists of pharmacy technicians working in remote locations, or pharmacist supervision of nurses performing pharmacy functions in small hospitals and nursing homes (Casey et al., 2001; Cooksey et al., 2002).

Mental and Behavioral Health Care Professionals

The bulk of mental and behavioral health services in rural areas are delivered by generalist physicians (Hartley et al., 1999). The specialists that provide these services, including psychiatrists (specialist physicians), clinical psychologists, counselors, social workers, and therapists with masters-level training are all in short supply in rural areas (Ivey et al., 1998).

Meeting the needs of rural communities for mental and behavioral health services will likely require a multifaceted approach. Cross-training of generalist physicians at rural training sites to facilitate screening, diagnosis, and referrals for mental health care would extend access to appropriate care in rural areas. Rural-focused residency programs in psychiatry might be developed for specialist physicians as well. Another option is to train more midlevel clinicians to provide mental and behavioral health services. For example, some success has been achieved in training advanced practice psychiatric nurses as either clinical nurse specialists (oriented toward psychotherapy) or psychiatric nurse practitioners (oriented toward the physiological bases of disease and case management). Nine rural states currently have degree programs (master's or doctoral) in advanced practice psychiatric nursing, and the curricula of these programs target the identification and treatment of the chronically mentally ill (Hartley et al., 2004). On the other hand, efforts to fill the need for mental health providers through expanded use of psychologists with master's degrees have encountered opposition from professional leadership within the field of psychology (see the discussion below of licensure and scope of practice).

Health Administrators

Few health administration programs train their students explicitly for careers in rural areas. Traditionally, many rural health administrators have backgrounds in clinical or technical fields and have learned management skills on the job (Robertson and Cockley, 2004). Competencies recently identified for rural health administration students highlight facility in adapting conventional management approaches to rural needs for health care (given the older age profile and specific health concerns of rural residents), an understanding of reimbursement mechanisms (in light of the greater reliance on public payers), and expertise in managing multidisciplinary teams and evaluating small organizations (to address the broad range of duties typically carried out by small numbers of staff as compared with urban sites) (Robertson and Cockley, 2004).

A recent survey of health administration programs sheds light on some of the opportunities to incorporate a rural focus into the curricula of master's-level programs (Reed and Hawkins, 2001). Over two-thirds of health administration programs are located in public institutions, where state legislatures could provide funding or other incentives for targeted rural training. The majority of programs are associated with health professions schools (e.g., public health, medicine, nursing, allied health), providing opportunities for cross-training and interdisciplinary approaches important to team work. To increase rural enrollment through place-based learning, more than a third have distance coursework, and nine offer distance degrees. Eighty percent require field experience (an average of 16 weeks) as part of their program.

Public Health Professionals

Several IOM reports have pointed to the need for significant improvement in the U.S. public health infrastructure in order to better serve the needs of population health (IOM, 2001, 2003b, 2004b). A competently trained workforce is an essential element of the public health infrastructure. The public health workforce at the federal, state, and local levels must be prepared to meet an array of needs, such as providing community health education and information dissemination, ensuring health-related environmental safety, and responding to community emergencies (IOM, 2003b; NACRHHS, 2000). In 2001, the Centers for Disease Control and Prevention (CDC) found that 80 percent of the existing public health workforce lacked any formal training (an exception to this rule may be nurses). As many rural areas are not near an educational institution or do not have a well-developed public health program, most local community public health employees have had to learn on the job (NACRHHS, 2000). This gap seriously compromises a community's ability to engage in surveillance activities necessary to prevent disease and maintain the health of the population.

Based on the findings of the 2001 survey, the CDC has called for public health departments to recruit and train new personnel. An earlier IOM committee recommended that such training programs take advantage of online education and interactive distance learning models to expand the education base (IOM, 2003b). Rural communities could establish innovative partnerships among local community colleges, schools of medicine and nursing, and public health departments to support educational requirements and lifelong learning (NACRHHS, 2000). These educational systems might be founded on the competency sets identified by the IOM (2003b):

- *Core*—basic skills needed to perform the essential functions of public health
    - *Function-specific*—leadership, management, supervisory, support staff
    - *Discipline-specific*—community dentistry, other professionals or technical specialists

- *Subject-specific*—maternal and child health, vaccine-preventable disease, cancer, chronic diseases
- *Workplace basics* (required of all personnel)—literacy, writing and presentation skills, and computer literacy

In addition, ensuring a public health workforce requires monitoring workforce composition and future needs and developing curricula to meet these needs, implementing incentives to promote population health practices, conducting and supporting evaluation and research of population health, and sustaining financial support for learning systems (IOM, 2003b).

Recruitment and Retention

The health care workforce of rural communities is dependent on the ability to both recruit and retain trained health professionals. The primary focus of federal and state policy has been on recruitment, with much less emphasis on retention.

Recruitment

HRSA and 41 states (1996 data) sponsor both loan repayment and scholarship programs that bring hundreds of new health professionals to rural areas under multiyear service commitments (Hart et al., 2002). The National Health Service Corps (NHSC) is perhaps the best recognized of these programs, placing primary care providers, dentists, and mental health providers (both physicians and nonphysicians) in designated health professions shortage areas, often at federally supported clinics. NHSC has yet to yield a predictable supply of physicians for rural areas because enrollment depends on the numbers of graduating students with an interest in primary care and because medical school debt places strong financial pressure on graduates (Mueller, 2002). Federal Title VII and VIII health professions training programs have a broader scope than NHSC, encompassing the training of physicians, nurses, dentists, pharmacists, and public health and allied health professionals (NRHA, 2004).

States and regions also facilitate rural placement using recruitment databases, such as the Iowa Health Professions Inventory; the Southern Rural Access Program, which recruits primary care providers for 8 southern states; and the National Rural Recruitment and Retention Network, in which 37 states participate (Gamm et al., 2003; WHA, 2004). Federally designated shortage areas (including health professions shortage areas for primary health care, dental care, and mental health, and medically underserved areas) are eligible to offer both federal and state scholarship and loan repayments, as well as to participate in related HRSA workforce programs including NHSC. Lack of data on the numbers of health professionals in rural areas hampers the process of designation and assignment, however, as well as the efficient use of scarce resources. In the case of mental health, for example, states may count either psychiatrists only, or other mental health specialists as well (i.e., social workers, clinical psychologists, clinical social workers, and therapists), in proposing that a county or locality be designated as a shortage area. Because few data are available on the numbers of nonpsychiatrist specialists actually involved in clinical practice and their hours, their specialties, and their practice sites, many states opt to rely on existing information on the number of psychiatrists—typically few or none in rural communities. The potential capacity of nonpsychiatrists may be underestimated as a result, and thus it becomes difficult or impossible to target behavioral health resources appropriately to those areas most in need.

International medical graduates (IMGs) are another source of physicians for many rural areas. Nationally, IMGs make up almost one-quarter of the nation's supply of physicians actively involved in patient care in both urban and rural areas (2001 data, as cited in Hart et al., 2002). Despite potential mismatches between the skills of IMGs (who are often subspecialty trained in urban research-affiliated settings) and local needs for primary care, as well as a retention rate of about 50 percent after 3 years (the length of the typical service obligation), IMGs are commonly found in rural critical access hospitals in counties defined as persistently poor and in some of the most remote and smallest hospitals (Hagopian et al., 2004; WHA, 2004). IMGs are also hired by hospitals as specialists to fill critical general surgery, radiology, and anesthesiology vacancies (Mueller, 2002).

Despite their importance in certain underserved rural areas, IMGs may not be a reliable source in the future because of tightened security following the September 11 terrorist attacks (Mueller, 2002). It would be difficult to replace all waiver physicians with domestic medical school graduates. To replace the 727 new J-1 waiver physicians who entered the workforce in 2000, rural areas would need to recruit one-sixth of all domestic medical school graduates with primary care training, over and above the 365 NHSC physicians and all others already practicing in the area of primary care.

Retention

To enhance retention, many steps have been taken to address key concerns of rural clinicians. There have been few evaluations of such programs, however, so little is known about the impact of different approaches.

Even when salaries are roughly comparable between rural and urban areas, as is the case for generalist and specialist physicians, rural providers tend to work more hours per week, see larger numbers of patients, and have greater demands for on-call coverage (Hart et al., 2002; Williams et al., 2001). To compensate rural providers more equitably and improve recruitment and retention, the federal and some state governments provide higher payments to physicians in some rural areas. The Medicare program offers a 10 percent supplemental payment to physicians practicing in rural areas designated as health professions shortage areas, an incentive made automatic under the Medicare Modernization Act of 2003. In addition, the act includes a new 5 percent bonus payment to physicians in designated scarcity areas (in terms of either primary care or the availability of specialists) effective from 2005 through 2007 (Hart et al., 2002; MedPAC, 2004). In a similar vein, the Utah Medicaid program has improved recruitment and retention of dentists through a 20 percent reimbursement incentive (Gordon, 2004).

Incentives for building a rural practice are also a part of federal programs for community health centers and rural health clinics. Providers may qualify for supplemental grants or higher reimbursement rates through the Centers for Medicare and Medicaid Services. For example, community health centers receive federal grants covering the cost of primary care and support services (e.g., transportation, translation) for low-income people living in medically underserved areas (Bloom et al., 2001). Rural health clinics do not qualify for grants, but can receive cost-based reimbursement for care provided by a number of midlevel clinicians.

In an effort to address the heavy workload and on-call burden of rural clinicians, some rural communities take advantage of either locum tenums programs, which offer respite and backup for providers in remote areas, or temporary contracts with provider groups (an alternative to locum tenums often used by hospitals in need of emergency medical services backup) (Williams et al., 2001). Under the auspices of The Robert Wood Johnson Foundation's Practice Sites Program during the mid-1990s, for example, state health departments in Nebraska and New Mexico created innovative locum tenums networks (RWJF, 2000a,b). These respite programs also provide an opportunity for health professionals to partake periodically of cer-

---

BOX 4-2
Mansfield University Master's Program
in Community Psychology

From 1977 until 2000, Mansfield University, a public institution in rural north-central Pennsylvania, offered a master's degree in community psychology (Murray and Keller, 1998). This program recruited many of its students from rural areas; exposed students to rural issues through course curricula; trained them at rural sites under the supervision of faculty extensively involved in local concerns; and placed them in rural jobs, many in public agencies in Pennsylvania and neighboring New York. Closure of the program reflected a number of considerations: difficulty in recruiting qualified students, insufficient funding support and pressure from the state higher educational system to cut smaller programs, and lack of authorization from the state to offer doctoral training at a time when Pennsylvania was joining many other states in requiring doctoral-level training for clinical psychologists.

---

tain cultural and social aspects of urban environments, and this may be particularly important for those who are not from rural environments.

State licensure and scope-of-practice statutes can impede or facilitate the flow of health professionals into rural areas by influencing both the roles played by different types of health professionals and the financial playing field (i.e., eligibility for reimbursement of certain services under public and private insurance programs). Given that rural areas are far more dependent than urban on midlevel clinicians, licensure and scope-of-practice laws can have a sizable impact on the rural workforce.

Some states allow for a broader scope of practice for midlevel clinicians and for long-distance (rather than on-site) supervision by physicians and other specialists (Hartley et al., 2002). In the case of mental health, for example, most rural states have granted prescribing authority to advanced practice psychiatric nurses (Gamm and Hutchison, 2004). A few pilot studies have found positive outcomes of expanded scope of practice for dental hygienists, although most states do not permit them independent practice (Nolan et al., 2003). There have also been recent examples of professional groups and states tightening licensure requirements or narrowing the scope of practice for some types of midlevel clinicians, such as master's-level psychologists (see Box 4-2). Moreover, as discussed in Chapter 5, payment policies can hamper recruitment of providers if they fail to recognize the mix and complement of providers available to deliver services in rural areas.

It is beyond the scope of this report to speak to the minimum educational requirements for licensure or the appropriate scopes of practice for various types of health care professionals, but it is important to note that the decisions of professional organizations and state governments on these matters have an important impact on the rural workforce. The committee does emphasize that decisions regarding licensure and scope of practice will best serve the needs of the population if they are grounded in strong evidence on the quality of care provided by various types of health care professionals. The current evidence base is very lean, and research in this area would thus be a highly worthwhile investment.

Continuing education, whether delivered on site or remotely, provides opportunities for enhanced training, reduces professional isolation, and increases collaboration within and across the health professions. EMS programs in Montana and New Mexico have used remote continuing education to retain rural health professionals while expanding the scope of practice for both licensed providers and paraprofessionals. For example, New Mexico's Red River Project has trained EMTs in triage and referral to primary care providers (Gamm et al., 2003; NRHA, 1997).

Lastly, recruitment and retention of health care professionals will likely improve to the extent that rural hospitals and other provider organizations exhibit the key characteristics associated with enhanced staff satisfaction and professional development. For example, key characteristics of "magnet hospitals," hospitals that have exhibited success in recruitment and retention of nurses, include participatory management style, able and qualified leaders at each level of the organization (both nursing and nonnursing leaders), and executive-level nursing leadership with decentralized department structures (McClure and Hinshaw, 2002).

OPTIONS FOR MOBILIZING COMMUNITY RESOURCES

As discussed in Chapter 2, maximizing both individual and population health requires the active engagement of the entire population. Health care professionals have an important role to play, but so do the residents of a community. There is also a need for strong leadership and collaboration to muster communitywide resources in support of efforts to improve health and health care.

Evidence suggests that major improvements in the health status of the population will most likely be achieved by a shift in emphasis from treatment to prevention of disease. Behavior and environment are responsible for more than 70 percent of avoidable mortality (McGinnis and Foege, 1993). Health care is important, but it is just one of several determinants of health (McGinnis et al., 2002).

The residents of a community make both individual and collective decisions that influence the incidence and prevalence of disease. Individual behaviors (e.g., diet, exercise, tobacco and alcohol consumption) have been linked to the emergence and progression of most if not all leading health conditions, including heart disease, diabetes, asthma, and cancer. Health is also shaped by laws and policies, employment and income, and social norms and other factors that influence individual behaviors and environmental conditions that undermine health (McGinnis et al., 2002).

Residents play an important role as well in the ongoing management of chronic conditions. Chronic conditions are long-term, frequently require ongoing care, and often limit what the individual can do. People with such conditions often see many clinicians in different care settings and must possess certain skills to navigate the health system successfully. Advice from health care providers can be conflicting, and drug–drug interactions are common (Classen, 1999). Self-care is critical to the management of many chronic conditions, as well as care provided by family and friends on which many people with chronic conditions rely (Van Korff et al., 1997).

Health literacy influences the likelihood that an individual will pursue a healthy lifestyle, interact effectively with the health care system, and engage actively in the ongoing management of chronic conditions. Health literacy skills are needed to read and understand health information (e.g., immunization schedules, drug inserts, hospital discharge instructions); to calculate the timing and dosage of medicines; to evaluate and make decisions about treatment options and participation in clinical trials; to understand and give consent (e.g., complete an advance directive); and to navigate the health care system effectively (IOM, 2004b). Health literacy is influenced by three factors (IOM, 2004b):

- *Education system*—Nearly one-half of all adults (or 90 million individuals) in the United States have limited functional literacy skills, where literacy is defined as a basic set of reading, writing, mathematics, speech, and speech comprehension skills (Kirsch, 2001).
- *Health system*—A large body of evidence (more than 300 publications) indicates that most health-related materials far exceed the average reading ability of U.S. adults.
- *Culture and society*—The shared ideas, meanings, and values of the

residents of a community give significance to health information and messages, shape perceptions of health and illness, and influence the use of the health care system.

As discussed above, enhancements of precollegiate education aimed at ensuring an adequate pool of rural students prepared to pursue health professions careers will likely contribute to increased literacy and health literacy on the part of the general population. But greater emphasis on science and health education will not be enough. Raising population-wide literacy and health literacy will require much broader improvements in grade K through 12 education.

Within the purview of the health system, a great deal can be done to improve health literacy. As recommended in an earlier IOM report (IOM, 2004b), health care providers, purchasers, and other stakeholders should improve their health-related communications by engaging consumers in the development of health messages, exploring creative approaches to the communication of health information using printed and electronic materials and media, and establishing methods for creating health information content in appropriate and clear language. The report also recommends that cultural and linguistic competency of health care providers be included as an essential measure of the quality of care, and that public and private oversight, accreditation, and certification programs incorporate health literacy into their standards for health care professionals and organizations.

As discussed in Chapter 6, expansion of access to the Internet and establishment of a National Health Information Infrastructure open up many opportunities to enhance health communication and provide a variety of other supports to residents of rural communities. Indeed, the focus of informatics is shifting from provider-oriented to consumer-oriented information and decision support (see Figure 4-2).

This shift raises key issues that will need to be addressed in the coming years:

• How best to guide consumers to reliable and understandable sources of clinical and other information (e.g., scientific evidence, practice guidelines, best practices).

• What ICT tools will be most useful to consumers in managing their own health (e.g., personal health records, web-based support groups).

• What steps can be taken now to better prepare the lay public to interact with and derive the greatest benefit from the ICT resources that are steadily becoming available in most communities.

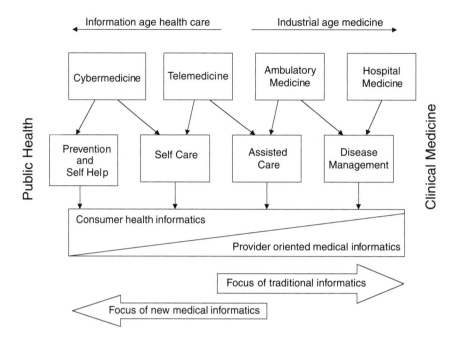

FIGURE 4-2 The focus of traditional medical informatics is shifting from health professionals to consumers.
SOURCE: Eysenbach, 2000.

Now is the time for all communities, both rural and urban, to begin preparing for the dramatic changes in health and health care that are likely to occur in the coming decade. As they go down this road, communities will be able to learn a great deal from each other, as well as from efforts under way in other countries (Detmer et al., 2003).

CONCLUSIONS AND RECOMMENDATIONS

Human resources—both health care professionals and the population at large in the community—are critical assets in every rural community's efforts to improve both individual and population health. The current health care workforce, including that in rural areas, is poorly prepared to address the quality challenge. Most formal educational programs for health professionals place limited emphasis on the core competencies identified by the IOM (2003c). Existing workforce training programs using supportive information technology should be strengthened to assist health care professionals already in practice in mastering these competencies.

> **Recommendation 3. Congress should provide appropriate resources to the Health Resources and Services Administration to expand experientially based workforce training programs in rural areas to ensure that all health care professionals master the core competencies of providing patient-centered care, working in interdisciplinary teams, employing evidence-based practice, applying quality improvement, and utilizing informatics. These competencies are relevant to the many discipline-specific and multidisciplinary programs supported under Titles VII and VIII of the Social Security Act.**

There are many opportunities to redesign existing workforce training programs in ways that will support rural communities in their efforts to improve the quality of health care and enhance population health:

• More stable and generous funding should be provided for the Quentin Burdick Program to conduct demonstrations in several rural communities. These demonstrations should provide for (1) the training of leadership teams to mobilize community resources, (2) communitywide health literacy programs, and (3) interdisciplinary health professions education in the core competencies essential to improving quality.

• Workforce programs such as HRSA's Area Health Education Centers, Health Education and Training Centers, and Geriatric Education Centers should explicitly target rural localities, and broaden their scope beyond physician supply to include midlevel providers in specialties in short supply in rural areas (e.g., mental health and substance abuse and emergency care).

• Workforce programs that recruit students from minority and underserved communities for health professions careers in rural communities—such as the Health Careers Opportunity Program, HRSA's Centers of Excellence program, scholarship and loan repayment programs for disadvantaged students, and such programs offered by IHS—should expand their recruitment and placement efforts in rural communities.

In expanding experientially based workforce recruitment and training programs, the federal government should place particular emphasis on the types of health professionals that are in very short supply and on the geographic areas experiencing the greatest difficulty in recruitment and retention. Current workforce programs are hampered by a lack of data and information to target resources effectively.

> *Key Finding 3. To target workforce training programs most effectively, federal, state, and local governments need better information on the current supply and types of health professionals. Data that would be particularly useful include the numbers of providers and provider hours of clinical practice, practice specialties, and sites of service. Financial and policy incentives at the federal and state levels could be put in place to facilitate the gathering, analysis, and retention of health professions workforce data that are comparable across states.*

Enhancing experientially based workforce training programs is an important first step, but it will not be enough. Fundamental change in health professions education programs will be needed to produce an adequate supply of properly educated health care professionals for rural and frontier communities. A multifaceted approach to the recruitment and retention of health professionals in rural areas is needed, including interventions at every point along the rural workforce pipeline: (1) enhanced preparation of rural elementary and high school students to pursue health careers; (2) stronger commitment of health professions education programs to recruiting students from rural areas, educating and training students in those areas, and adopting rural-appropriate curricula; and (3) a variety of strong incentives for health professionals to seek and retain employment in rural communities. To achieve the goal of an adequate and sustained supply of health care providers in rural areas, it will be necessary to undertake interventions at all of these points and to do so in a coordinated fashion.

Enhancements to the basic curriculum, particularly the science curriculum, for middle and high school students are needed to better prepare rural students for careers in the health professions. HRSA's Office of Rural Health Policy could work collaboratively with the various federal agencies (e.g., Bureau of Health Professions, Department of Education, Bureau of Indian Affairs, and IHS), professional associations, and rural constituencies to identify enhancements to the basic curriculum, particularly the science curriculum, for middle and high school students that would better prepare them for rural careers in the health professions. A rural health professions mentoring program might be established to expose rural students to potential careers in health care.

Changes are also needed in health professions education programs. Greater effort must be made to recruit students from rural areas, to locate a meaningful portion of the formal educational experience in rural settings, and to develop education programs that are relevant to rural practice.

Recommendation 4. Schools of medicine, dentistry, nursing, allied health, and public health and programs in mental and behavioral health should:

- **Work collaboratively to establish outreach programs to rural areas to attract qualified applicants.**
- **Locate a meaningful portion of the educational experience in rural communities. Universities and 4-year colleges should expand distance learning programs and/or pursue formal arrangements with community and other colleges, including tribal and traditionally African American colleges, located in rural areas to extend the array of rural-based education options while encouraging students to pursue higher levels of education.**
- **Make greater effort to recruit faculty with experience in rural practice, and develop rural-relevant curricula addressing areas that are key to improving health and health care, including the five core competencies (i.e., providing patient-centered care, working in interdisciplinary teams, employing evidence-based practice, applying quality improvement, and utilizing informatics), the fundamentals of population health, and leadership skills.**
- **Develop rural training tracks and fellowships that (1) provide students with rotations in rural provider sites; (2) emphasize primary care practice; and (3) provide cross-training in key areas of shortage in rural communities, such as emergency and trauma care, mental health, and obstetrics.**

Furthermore, the federal government should provide financial incentives for residency training programs to provide rural tracks by linking some portion of the graduate medical education payments under Medicare to achievement of this goal.

The residents of rural communities also have a key role to play in improving population health. Residents can contribute to improving their own health and that of others by pursuing healthy behaviors and complying with treatment regimens, assuming appropriate caregiving roles for family members and neighbors, and volunteering for community health improvement efforts. In many rural populations, low levels of health literacy (the degree to which individuals have the capacity to obtain, process, and understand basic health information) currently hamper efforts to engage residents in health-related activities. The Department of Education and state education agencies should work in partnership with local nonprofit literacy associations and libraries to measure and improve the health literacy of rural community residents by, among other things, providing access to Internet-based health resources and training in information technology.

REFERENCES

AMA (American Medical Association). 2002. *State Medical Licensure Requirements and Statistics, 2001–2002.* [Online]. Available: http://www.ama-assn.org/ama/upload/mm/40/table14.pdf [accessed September 2004].

Baer LD, Smith LM. 1999. Nonphysician professionals and rural America. In: Ricketts T, ed. *Rural Health in the United States.* New York: Oxford University Press. Pp. 52–60.

BHPR (Bureau of Health Professions). 2004a. *Area Health Education Centers.* [Online]. Available: http://bhpr.hrsa.gov/ahec/ [accessed May 3, 2004].

BHPR. 2004b. *Diversity.* [Online]. Available: http://bhpr.hrsa.gov/diversity/default.htm [accessed July 20, 2004].

BHPR. 2004c. *Geriatric Education Training Centers.* [Online]. Available: http://bhpr.hrsa.gov/interdisciplinary/gec.html [accessed May 12, 2004].

BHPR. 2004d. *Health Education and Training Centers.* [Online]. Available: http://bhpr.hrsa.gov/interdisciplinary/hetc.html [accessed May 12, 2004].

BHPR. 2004e. *Public Health Traineeship.* [Online]. Available: http://bhpr.hrsa.gov/publichealth/phtrainee.htm [accessed August 9, 2004].

Biola H, Green LA, Phillips RL, Guirguis-Blake J, Fryer GE. 2003. The U.S. primary care physician workforce: Undervalued service. *American Family Physician* 68:1486.

Bloom D, Canning D, Sevilla J. 2001. *The Effect of Health on Economic Growth: Theory and Evidence.* New York: National Bureau of Economic Research.

Bodenheimer T, Lorig K, Holman H, Grumbach K. 2002a. Patient self-management of chronic disease in primary care. *Journal of the American Medical Association* 288(19):2469–2475.

Bodenheimer T, Wagner EH, Grumbach K. 2002b. Improving primary care for patients with chronic illness. *Journal of the American Medical Association* 288(14):1775–1779.

Buckwalter K. 2004. *Workforce: Training Deployment and Support.* Presentation at the Workshop on the Future of Rural Health: A Quality Focus (March 1–2, 2004). Washington, DC.

Casey M, Klingner J, Moscovice I. 2001 (July). *Access to Rural Pharmacy Services in Minnesota, North Dakota, and South Dakota.* Minneapolis, MN: Rural Health Research Center, University of Minnesota.

Classen DC. 1999. Adverse drug events and medication errors: The scientific perspective. In: *Enhancing Patient Safety and Reducing Errors.* Chicago, IL: National Patient Safety Foundation. Pp. 56–60.

Collins KS, Hughes DL, Doty MM, Ives BL, Edwards JN, Tenney K. 2002. *Diverse Communities, Common Concerns: Assessing Health Care Quality for Minority Americans.* New York: The Commonwealth Fund.

Cooksey JA, Knapp KK, Walton SM, Cultice JM. 2002. Challenges to the pharmacist profession from escalating pharmaceutical demand. *Health Affairs* 21(5):182–188.

Cooper LA, Roter DL, Johnson RL, Ford DE, Steinwachs DM, Powe NR. 2003. Patient-centered communication, ratings of care, and concordance of patient and physician race. *Annals of Internal Medicine* 139:907–915.

Detmer DE, Singleton PD, Macleod A, Wait S, Taylor M, Ridwell J. 2003 (March). *The Informed Patient: Study Report.* Cambridge, UK: Judge Institute of Management, Cambridge University Health.

Dezendorf PK, Scott RL. 2001. Using distance education to teach and manage a community health rotation in rural Appalachia. *Perspective on Physician Assistant Education* 12(4):255–258.

DiCenso A, Cullum N, Ciliska D. 1998. Implementing evidence-based nursing: Some misconceptions [editorial]. *Evidence-Based Nursing* 1:38–40.

Evers G. 2001. Naming nursing: Evidence-based nursing. *Nursing Diagnosis* 12(4):127–142.

Eysenbach G. 2000. Consumer health informatics. *British Medical Journal* 320:1713–1716.

Fos P, Hutchison L. 2003. The state of rural oral health. In: Gamm L, Hutchison L, Bellamy G, Dabney B, eds. *Rural Healthy People 2010.* Vol. 1. Pp. 199–203.

Franks PE, Kocher N, Chapman S. 2004. *Emergency Medical Technicians and Paramedics in California.* San Francisco, CA: The Center for the Health Professions.

French P. 1999. The development of evidence-based nursing. *Journal of Advanced Medicine* 29(1):72–78.

Gamm L, Hutchison L. 2004 (February). *Mental Health and Substance Abuse Services: Prospects for Rural Communities.* Commissioned Paper for the IOM Committee on the Future of Rural Health Care. Washington, DC.

Gamm L, Hutchison L, Bellamy G, Dabney B. 2002. Rural healthy people 2010: Identifying rural health priorities and models for practice. *Journal of Rural Health* 18(1):9–14.

Gamm L, Hutchison L, Dabney B, Dorsey A. 2003. *Rural Healthy People 2010: A Companion Document to Healthy People 2010.* Vol. 1. College Station, TX: Texas A&M University System Health Science Center, School of Rural Public Health, Southwest Rural Health Research Center.

Gordon D. 2004. *Rural Health Brief: Where Have All the Dentists Gone?* Washington, DC: National Conference of State Legislatures.

Grad R, Macauley AC, Warner M. 2001. Teaching evidence-based medical care: Description and evaluation. *Family Medicine* 33(8):602–606.

Hagopian A, Thompson MJ, Kaltenbach E, Hart LG. 2004. The role of international medical graduates in America's small rural critical access hospitals. *Journal of Rural Health* 20(1):52–58.

Hart LG, Salsberg E, Phillips DM, Lishner DM. 2002. Rural health care providers in the United States. *Journal of Rural Health* 18(Supplement):211–232.

Hart LG, Lishner DM, Rosenblatt RA. 2003. Rural health workforce: Context, trends, and issues. In: Larson EH, Johnson KE, Norris TE, Lishner DM, Rosenblatt RA, Hart LG, eds. *State of the Health Workforce in Rural America: Profiles and Comparisons.* Seattle, WA: WWAMI. Pp. 7–14.

Hartley D, Bird D, Dempsey P. 1999. Rural mental health and substance abuse. In: Ricketts TC, ed. *Rural Health in the United States.* New York: Oxford University Press. Pp. 159–178.

Hartley D, Ziller E, Lambert D, Loux S, Bird D. 2002 (October). *State Licensure Laws and the Mental Health Professions: Implications for the Rural Mental Health Workforce.* Portland, ME: Maine Rural Health Research Center.

Hartley D, Hart V, Hanrahan N, Loux S. 2004. *Are Advanced Practice Psychiatric Nurses a Solution to Rural Mental Health Workforce Shortages.* Portland, ME: Maine Rural Health Research Center.

Haynes RB. 2002. What kind of evidence is it that evidence-based medicine advocates want healthcare providers and consumers to pay attention to? *BMC Health Services Research* 2(1):3.

Hooker RB. 2002. Trends in the supply of physician assistants and nurse practitioners in the United States. *Health Affairs* 21(5):164–181.

HRSA (Health Resources and Services Administration). 2000. *The Pharmacist Workforce: A Study of the Supply and Demand for Pharmacists.* Rockville, MD: U.S. Department of Health and Human Services.

HRSA. 2004a. *Preview of FY2004 Funding Opportunities. Health Professions Education and Training Funding Opportunities.* [Online]. Available: http://www.hrsa.gov/grants/preview/professions.htm [accessed August 9, 2004].

HRSA. 2004b. *Preview of FY2004 Funding Opportunities. Rural Health Funding Opportunities.* [Online]. Available: http://www.hrsa.gov/grants/preview/rural.htm [accessed August 9, 2004].

HRSA. 2004c. *Preview of FY2005 Funding Opportunities. Loan Repayments and Scholarships.* [Online]. Available: http://www.hrsa.gov/grants/preview/ [accessed August 9, 2004].

IOM (Institute of Medicine). 2001. *Crossing the Quality Chasm: A New Health System for the 21st Century.* Washington, DC: National Academy Press.

IOM. 2003a. *Unequal Treatment: Confronting Racial and Ethnic Disparities in Health Care.* Washington, DC: The National Academies Press.

IOM. 2003b. *The Future of the Public's Health in the 21st Century.* Washington, DC: The National Academies Press.

IOM. 2003c. *Health Professions Education. A Bridge to Quality.* Washington, DC: The National Academies Press.

IOM. 2003d. *Keeping Patients Safe: Transforming the Work Environment for Nurses.* Washington, DC: The National Academies Press.

IOM. 2004a. *Academic Health Centers: Leading Change in the 21st Century.* Washington, DC: The National Academies Press.

IOM. 2004b. *Health Literacy: A Prescription to End Confusion.* Washington, DC: The National Academies Press.

IOM. 2004c. *In the Nation's Compelling Interest: Ensuring Diversity in the Health Care Workforce.* Washington, DC: The National Academies Press.

IOM. 2004d. *Patient Safety: Achieving a New Standard for Care.* Washington, DC: The National Academies Press.

Ivey SL, Scheffler R, Zazzali JL. 1998. Supply dynamics of the mental health workforce: Implications for health policy. *Milbank Quarterly* 76(1):25–28.

Jadad AB, Haynes RB. 1998. The Cochrane collaboration: Advances and challenges in improving evidence-based decision making. *Medical Decision Making* 1:2–9; discussion 16–18.

Johnson J. 2002. Partnerships for training impacts physician assistant education and practice in rural areas. *Perspective on Physician Assistant Education* 13(2):106–107.

Kirsch IS. 2001. *The International Adult Literacy Survey (IALS): Understanding What Was Measured.* Princeton, NJ: Educational Testing Service.

Lang NM. 1999. Discipline-based approaches to evidence-based practice: A view from nursing. Joint Commission. *Journal on Quality Improvement* 255(10):539–544.

Liederman EM, Morefield CS. 2003. Web messaging: A new tool for patient-physician communication. *Journal of the American Medical Informatics Association* 10(3):260–270.

Lorig KR, Sobel DS, Stewart AL, Brown BW Jr, Bandura A, Ritter P, Gonzalez VM, Laurent DD, Holman HR. 1999. Evidence suggesting that a chronic disease self-management program can improve health status while reducing hospitalization: A randomized trial. *Medical Care* 37(1):5–14.

Mazurek B. 2002. Strategies for overcoming barriers in implementing evidence-based practice. *Pediatric Nursing* 28(2):159–161.

McClure ML, Hinshaw, AS. 2002. *Magnet Hospitals Revisited: Attraction and Retention of Professional Nurses.* Washington, DC: American Nurses Publishing.

McGinnis MJ, Foege WH. 1993. Actual causes of death in the United States. *Journal of the American Medical Association* 270(18):2207–2212.

McGinnis MJ, Williams-Russo P, Knickman JR. 2002. The case for more active policy attention to health promotion. *Health Affairs* 21:78–93.

MedPAC (Medicare Payment Advisory Commission). 2004. *Report to Congress: Medicare Payment Policy.* Washington, DC: MedPAC.

Moorhead JC, Gallery ME, Hirshkorn C, Barnaby DP, Barsan WG, Conrad LC, Dalsey WC, Fried M, Herman SH, Hogan P, Mannle TE, Packard DC, Perina DG, Pollack CV Jr, Rapp MT, Rorrie CC Jr, Schafermeyer RW. 2002. A study of the workforce in emergency medicine. *Annals of Emergency Medicine* 40(1):3–18.

Mueller K. 2002. *The Immediate and Future Role of the J-1 Visa Waiver Program for Physicians: The Consequences of Change for Rural Health Care Service Delivery.* [Online]. Available: http://www.rupri.org/publications/archive/reports/P2002-3/P2002-3.pdf [accessed July 6, 2004].

Murray JD, Keller PA. 1998. *Training Master's Degree Psychologists for Rural Practice: An Update.* [Online]. Available: http://www.narmh.org/pages/trafour.html [accessed June 3, 2004].

Myers WW. 2000. Commentary: The federal role in rural graduate medical education initiatives. *Journal of Rural Health* 16(3):301–303.

NACRHHS (National Advisory Committee on Rural Health and Human Services). 2000. *Rural Public Health: Issues and Considerations.* Washington, DC: U.S. Department of Health and Human Services.

NACRHHS. 2004. *The 2004 Report to the Secretary: Rural Health and Human Service Issues.* Rockville, MD: DHHS.

Newhouse JP, Williams AP, Bennett BW, Schwartz WB. 1982. Where have all the doctors gone? *Journal of the American Medical Association* 247(17):2392–2396.

Nolan L, Kamoie B, Harvey J, Vaquerano L, Blake S, Chawla S, Levi J, Rosenbaum S. 2003. *The Effects of State Dental Practice Laws Allowing Alternative Models of Preventive Oral Health Care Delivery to Low Income Children.* Washington, DC: The George Washington University Center for Health Services Research and Policy.

NRC (National Research Council). 1996. *National Science Education Standards.* Washington, DC: National Academy Press.

NRC. 2002. *Learning and Understanding: Improving Advanced Study of Mathematics and Science in U.S. High Schools.* Washington, DC: The National Academies Press.

NRC. 2003. *What Is the Influence of the National Science Education Standards.* Washington, DC: The National Academies Press.

NRHA (National Rural Health Association). 1997. *Rural and Frontier Emergency Medical Services toward the Year 2000.* [Online]. Available: http://www.nrharural.org/pagefile/issuepapers/ipaper9.html [accessed April 12, 2004].

NRHA. 2003. *Policy Brief: Health Care Workforce Distribution and Shortage Issues in Rural America.* [Online]. Available: http://www.nrharural.org/dc/policybriefs/WorkforceBrief.pdf [accessed April 6, 2004].

NRHA. 2004. *Policy Brief: Health Professions: Title VII of the Public Health Service Act Reauthorization.* [Online]. Available: http://www.nrharural.org/dc/policybriefs/HlthPrfsns.pdf [accessed April 6, 2004].

Rabinowitz HK, Taylor RB. 2004. *Caring for the Country: Family Doctors in Small Rural Towns.* New York, NY: Springer-Verlag Telos.

Rabinowtiz HK, Diamond JJ, Markham FW, Paynter NP. 2001. Critical factors for designing programs to increase the supply and retention of rural primary care physicians. *Journal of the American Medical Association* 286(9):1041–1048.

Rawlinson C, Crews P. 2003. Access to Quality Health Services in Rural Areas—Emergency Medical Services: A Literature Review. In: Gamm L, Hutchison L, Dabney B, Dorsey A, eds. *Rural Healthy People 2010. Access to Quality Health Services in Rural Areas.* College Station, TX: Southwest Rural Health Research Center, Texas A&M University. Pp. 77–81.

Reed L, Hawkins, V. 2001. *AUPHA Survey of Health Services Administration Education 2000–2001.* Washington, DC: Association of University Programs in Health Administration.

Robertson R, Cockley DE. 2004. Competencies for rural health administrators. *Journal of Health Administration Education* 21(3):329–341.

Rosenthal MB, Zaslavsky AM, Newhouse JP. 2003. *The Geographic Distribution of Physician Revisited.* Boston, MA: Harvard School of Public Health, Harvard University.

Rosswurm MA, Larrabee JH. 1999. A model for change to evidence-based practice. *Image Journal of Nursing Scholarship* 31(4):317–322.

Rural EMS Initiative. 2000. *Fact Sheet 2. North Dakota EMS Providers' Demographic and Work Characteristics.* Grand Forks, ND: University of North Dakota Center for Rural Health, School of Medicine and Health Sciences.

RWJF (The Robert Wood Johnson Foundation). 2000a. *National Program Project Report. Nebraska Practice Sites.* [Online]. Available: http://www.rwjf.org/reports/grr/028753.htm [accessed April 19, 2004].

RWJF. 2000b. *National Program Project Report. New Mexico Practice Sites.* [Online]. Available: http://www.rwjf.org/reports/grr/024627.htm [accessed April 19, 2004].

Scott D, Neary T, Thilliander T, Ueda C. 1992. Factors affecting pharmacists' selection of rural or urban practice sites in Nebraska. *American Journal of Hospital Pharmacy* 49:1941–1945.

Tooke-Rawlins D. 2000. Rural osteopathic family physician supply: Past and present. *Journal of Rural Health* 16(3):299–300.

USAC (Universal Service Administrative Company). 2004. *About RHCD.* [Online]. Available: http://www.rhc.universalservice.org/overview/rhcd.asp [accessed September 14, 2004].

USDHHS (Department of Health and Human Services). 2000. *Healthy People 2010: Understanding and Improving Health.* Washington, DC: Government Printing Office.

Van Korff M, Gruman J, Schaefer J, Curry SJ, Wagner EH. 1997. Collaborative management of chronic illness. *Annals of Internal Medicine* 127(12):1097–1102.

Walshe K, Rundall TG. 2001. Evidence-based management: From theory to practice in health care. *Milbank Quarterly* 70(3):429–457, IV–V.

WHA (Wisconsin Hospital Association). 2004. *Who Will Care for Our Patients? Wisconsin Takes Action to Fight a Growing Physician Shortage.* Madison, WI: Task Force on Wisconsin's Future Physician Workforce.

Williams JM, Ehrlich PF, Prescott JE. 2001. Emergency medical care in rural America. *Annals of Emergency Medicine* 38(3):323–327.

5

Finance

SUMMARY

The Quality Chasm *report calls for the implementation of payment systems that encourage the delivery of quality health care. This chapter begins by addressing how pay-for-performance initiatives should be implemented in rural communities. The committee recommends that rural demonstration projects be carried out to test different approaches to pay-for-performance systems in rural areas.*

To establish the right environment for the implementation of pay-for-performance initiatives, financial stability for rural health care delivery systems is required. Such stability is also required to finance investments in human resource networks and information and communications technology. Many rural health care delivery systems have been financially unstable. The chapter addresses the significant policy steps, most recently the Medicare Modernization Act of 2003, taken to address underpayment to rural providers. The committee believes it will be important to establish that these financial gains are being maintained.

In addition, major shortages of mental health and substance abuse professionals were documented earlier in this report. On the basis of these shortages, the committee concluded that a major assessment of the funding of mental health and substance abuse services in rural areas is required.

This chapter addresses rural health care finance in three broad areas. The first section examines pay-for-performance as a strategy for improving the quality of health care, as recommended in the *Quality Chasm* report (IOM, 2001). The second section reviews the various mechanisms used to fund rural health care services generally, while the third focuses on the special case of the funding of rural mental health and substance abuse services. The final section presents conclusions and recommendations.

PAY-FOR-PERFORMANCE

There is now a large evidence base, as documented in the *Quality Chasm* report (IOM, 2001) and discussed in Chapter 3, to substantiate a sizable gap between the health care services people receive and the services they should receive based on acknowledged best practices. To encourage providers to improve quality, some private and public purchasers have begun implementing a key recommendation of the *Quality Chasm* report: to link payments to measures of performance.

Because this is a relatively new strategy, there is only limited evidence available on the effects of pay-for-performance programs on quality. The Stanford University and University of California-San Francisco Evidence-based Practice Center, funded by the Agency for Healthcare Research and Quality, has just completed a literature review to identify published randomized controlled trials of incentive systems (Dudley et al., 2004). Of 5,045 publications reviewed, only 9 report results of randomized controlled trials on incentive systems. Of these 9 studies, 8 involved using specific financial incentives as interventions and tested a total of 10 hypotheses (Christensen et al., 1999; Davidson et al., 1992; Fairbrother et al., 2001; Hickson et al., 1987; Hillman et al., 1998, 1999; Kouides et al., 1998; Roski et al., 2003). In 6 cases, the incentive being tested was associated with the desired and statistically significant changes in the delivery of quality care, while in the other 4 cases, there was no significant difference in outcome between the control and the incentive arms of the trial. The remaining study involved reputational incentives as the intervention (Hibbard et al., 2003). In this study, hospitals with low performance scores that were released to the public were significantly more likely to engage in quality improvement activities than hospitals with high performance scores that were released to the public.

In summary, pay-for-performance research carried out using randomized controlled trials has produced some positive results. Some of the above trials demonstrated that introducing incentives can lead to desired improvements in the quality of care delivered. However, the scope of this research is still highly limited. The circumstances in which pay-for-performance techniques will succeed are not well understood. Further, 7 of the above 9 trials focused on the use of incentives to improve preventive care. Pay-for-performance incentives for a broader range of types of care need to be investigated.

Major Ongoing Pay-for-Performance Studies

Both private- and public-sector payers are now funding some major pay-for-performance studies. These are described in the following subsections.

Bridges to Excellence

Bridges to Excellence is a General Electric–led employer group initiative[1] aimed at improving the quality of care by recognizing and rewarding health care providers who demonstrate that they have implemented comprehensive solutions in managing their patients and deliver safe, effective, patient-centered, timely, efficient, and equitable care (Bridges to Excellence, 2003). The initiative encompasses three programs:

- *Physician Office Link*—Based on their implementation of specific processes to reduce errors and increase quality, physicians can earn up to $50 per year for each patient covered by a participating employer or plan.
- *Diabetes Care Link*—Enables physicians to achieve 1-year or 3-year recognition for high-quality care, with qualifying physicians receiving an $80 bonus for each diabetic patient covered by a participating employer or plan.
- *Cardiac Care Link*—Enables physicians to achieve 3-year recognition for high-quality care, with qualifying physicians eligible to receive up to $160 for each cardiac patient covered by a participating employer and plan.

Rewarding Results

A national initiative of The Robert Wood Johnson Foundation and the California HealthCare Foundation, Rewarding Results aims to invent, prove,

---

[1] Bridges to Excellence participants include large employers and health plans plus other organizations (including the Centers for Medicare and Medicaid Services, the National Committee for Quality Assurance, the Joint Commission on Accreditation of Healthcare Organizations, and the National Quality Forum) responsible for selecting, collecting, and reporting the measures.

and diffuse innovations in systems of provider payment and nonfinancial incentives that will encourage and reward high-quality health care. The foundations are awarding grants to plan, implement, and evaluate demonstrations of such provider payment systems and nonfinancial incentives (Rewarding Results, 2002).

National Voluntary Hospital Reporting Initiative

In December 2002, the American Hospital Association, Federation of American Hospitals, and Association of American Medical Colleges launched this initiative to collect and report hospital quality performance information (CMS, 2004a). The associations identified three conditions (acute myocardial infarction, heart failure, and pneumonia) for which they selected 10 measures. The Centers for Medicare and Medicaid Services (CMS) displays the data submitted by hospitals (www.cms.hhs.gov/quality/hospital). By February 2004, more than 1,400 hospitals were providing data on at least one of the measures (CMS, 2004a). Rural hospitals (excluding critical access hospitals) are participating in the study. To encourage participation, Section 501(b) of the Medicare Modernization Act of 2003 mandates that a hospital not submitting performance data for the 10 measures receive a 0.4 percent lower increase in prices for fiscal year 2005 than a hospital submitting such data.

Premier Hospital Quality Incentive Demonstration Project

Hospitals participating in the joint Premier, Inc.-CMS demonstration project will be eligible for increased Medicare payments if they are among the top performers in one of five clinical areas—heart attack, coronary artery bypass graft, heart failure, community-acquired pneumonia, and hip and knee replacement. The top 10 percent of hospitals in each clinical area will receive a 2 percent increase in Medicare payments; the next 10 percent will receive a 1 percent increase. Within the five areas, CMS will evaluate hospital performance on 34 measures, which include process steps, such as prompt administration of beta blockers, and outcomes, such as mortality rate. In the third year, participating hospitals that have failed to improve their performance in a specific clinical area beyond a minimum threshold established in the first year of the project will be subject to a payment reduction of 1 or 2 percent (CMS, 2004b). Premier, Inc., has announced that 278 hospitals have signed up for the project (Premier, Inc., 2003), 30 percent of which are rural hospitals, including some critical access hospitals (Personal communication, S. Alexander, May 27, 2004).

Pay-for-Performance Program Mandated in the Medicare Modernization Act of 2003

Section 649 of the Medicare Modernization Act of 2003 mandates that the Secretary of Health and Human Services establish a pay-for-performance demonstration program incorporating health information technology and evidence-based outcome measures. A maximum of four sites is mandated: two in urban areas; one in a rural area; and one in a state housing a medical school with a department of geriatrics that manages rural outreach sites and is capable of serving patients with multiple chronic conditions, one of which is dementia.

Challenges Facing Rural Providers

Even if payment for services is considered adequate by payer and provider alike, additional challenges remain for any effort to incorporate performance measures into payment calculations.

First, to the extent that an initiative to pay for performance requires investment in new information systems, other equipment, or additional personnel, rural providers are unlikely to have the reserves or borrowing capacity to provide that capital. Even when the capital is available, most rural providers must apply it to meeting their basic needs: new physical plant and equipment required for basic patient services. For example, many of the nation's rural hospitals were built during an era when inpatient care was the predominant mode of delivering services and before many changes were made in organizing even that form of care. These hospitals need to be modernized so they can be used as outpatient facilities and be more efficient providers of inpatient care.

A second challenge will be providers' natural proclivity to avoid any risk to their financial well-being—losing either dollars per service or total services. The threats to urban providers of thin or negative margins and losing patient business are too real to be set aside. Those providers in the most precarious financial position will require special consideration. In the most vulnerable places, where patient revenues in the best of circumstances are unlikely to be sufficient to sustain services, subsidies and investments in the tools needed for quality improvement are required (Mueller et al., 2003).

The source of the subsidy could also be the source of investment in quality initiatives designed to improve performance. For example, the Bureau of Primary Health Care has created a special grant program, Health Disparities Collaboratives: Changing Practice, Changing Lives, to achieve rapid improvements in the care provided through community health centers across the country, including those in rural areas. This example highlights the need for external investment in certain rural settings, as well as opportunities to fund that investment.

A further challenge in rural areas is one of scale. Measuring performance requires sufficient data to understand incidents in the context of processes of care in systems of health care delivery. As discussed earlier, conducting such analysis in a site that has a very limited number of possible encounters of interest (such as hospital admissions for particular conditions) can yield a distorted picture of the quality of care. To overcome this challenge, data can be aggregated across like providers in similar delivery systems to increase the number of patient encounters for which quality outcomes can be determined.

Pay-for-Performance Objectives, Approaches, and Measures

To date, pay-for-performance programs have focused primarily on encouraging providers to make changes in their own health care practices that will improve the quality of care for their patients. The committee believes that rural areas provide an opportunity to experiment with pay-for-performance strategies designed to encourage improvements in both individual practices and the overall community health system. Eventually, those demonstrations might be expanded even further to reward improvements in community health status, thus encouraging health care leaders to work collaboratively with other community leaders from educational institutions, social service agencies, and places of employment to achieve such improvement.

In sum, then, pay-for-performance incentives should seek to improve the quality of care delivered to individual patients and ultimately to raise the overall health status of the community. In particular, they should seek to encourage:

- Health care providers to make changes in their own practices that will improve the quality of care for individual patients.
- Health care providers to develop stronger collaborative relationships with each other to provide comprehensive, coordinated care where appropriate, for example, for chronically ill patients.

- Patients and their families to identify and demand high-quality care.
- The development of communitywide initiatives aimed at improving health behaviors.

Several financial approaches, possibly in combination, are available to achieve the above objectives:

- Giving providers higher payments for higher performance on quality measures.
- Requiring the payment of lower cost-sharing amounts and copayments if patients go to higher-quality providers as identified through quality measures.
- Sharing the savings from quality improvements between providers and patients.
- Employing risk sharing and capitation—payment mechanisms that provide incentives for better overall management of care across settings and time.

An important and difficult aspect of designing an incentive program is identifying appropriate measures of performance. Chapter 3 provides a detailed discussion of quality and quality measures. For each condition or group of conditions, a balanced set of measures is needed addressing the six quality aims set forth in the *Quality Chasm* report: safety, effectiveness, patient-centeredness, timeliness, efficiency, and equity (IOM, 2001). Further, measures are required for both individual and population health. In crafting these measures, consideration must be given to the cost and difficulty of applying them; standardization of measures will be helpful in this regard. Particularly important in the context of the present report is that the chosen measures must be capable of being applied to rural health care systems. Meeting this need may require addressing certain methodological issues; for example, small numbers for each facility may call for pooling of facilities.

Nearly all pay-for-performance experimentation is sponsored by health plans (Rosenthal et al., 2004) that serve primarily urban areas. The committee believes that there should be much greater pay-for-performance experimentation in rural areas than is currently planned and that there should be five pay-for-performance demonstration projects in rural communities—significantly more than the maximum of two mandated by the Medicare Modernization Act of 2003. These projects should be built around existing rural groupings of health care providers, for example, of rural health clinics, community health centers, and critical access hospitals. There should also be a demonstration project involving the linkage of several types of health care providers, such as hospitals, community health centers, and nursing homes. Finally, the payment methods tested should include both patient-based and community-based measures.

The pay-for-performance demonstration projects could also include incentives for using innovative ways of reducing waste. For example, in the delivery of primary care, potential savings might be derived from e-visits, group visits, and less-costly ways of handling chronic illness.

THE FUNDING OF RURAL HEALTH CARE

Significant proportions of the $1.55 trillion spent on health care in the United States in 2002 were spent on hospital care (31.3 percent), physician and clinical services (21.9 percent), dental services (4.5 percent), and nursing home and home health care (9.0 percent)[2] (Levit et al., 2004). In 2000, 1.3 percent of the total health care expenditure ($17 billion) was devoted to public health (Frist, 2002).

The financing of health care requires both payments for goods and services and capital for investment. Sources of payment for goods and services are both private (e.g., private insurance and direct patient payment) and public (e.g., public insurance programs such as Medicare and Medicaid, as well as federal, state, and local taxes). There are three sources of capital: the reserves providers accumulate, debt financing, and philanthropy.

Many types of health care providers in rural areas are highly dependent on Medicare and Medicaid for payment for services, and in some instances much more so than their urban counterparts. It has proven problematic to adapt the Medicare Prospective Payment System mandated in 1983 for inpatient hospital payments and in 1997 for outpatient and other services to the special circumstances of rural health. In some cases, the Prospective Payments System has led to underfunding of rural care. Moreover, recent stresses on state budgets have led to pressures to cut Medicaid rates and to restrict eligibility for the benefits, thereby reducing revenues for rural health care providers.

---

[2] Other major spending items are retail sales of medical products (mainly prescription drugs) (13.7 percent of the total), other professional services (3.0 percent of the total), other personal health care (2.9 percent of the total), administrative costs (6.8 percent of the total), and investment (3.7 percent of the total).

This section addresses the rural aspects of Medicare payments to hospitals and primary care physicians, as well as the funding of rural health clinics, community health centers, dental services, nursing homes, home health services, emergency medical services, and public health services. Weak financial performance by rural hospitals impacts their ability to raise capital, and this issue is addressed in the final subsection.

Medicare Hospital Payments

As suggested above, hospitals in rural areas (see Appendix C for an overview) are particularly dependent on Medicare funds. In 1999 Medicare paid 45 percent of total costs in rural hospitals as compared with 34 percent for their urban counterparts (MedPAC, 2001). Among rural hospitals, Medicare accounted for 60 percent of inpatient days in 1999, and for those hospitals with fewer than 50 beds, the proportion rose to 63 percent (Moscovice and Davidson, 2003).

Over the years since 1983, concerns about whether rural hospitals could survive under the Prospective Payment System have led Congress to create special categories of rural hospitals that receive either cost-based payments or elevated Prospective Payment System payments: rural referral centers, sole community hospitals, Medicare-dependent hospitals, and, most recently, community access hospitals. Notwithstanding these adjustments, throughout the 1990s inpatient Medicare margins for rural hospitals were substantially below urban margins. In the early 1990s, Medicare inpatient aggregate margins[3] were negative for both urban and rural hospitals. In the mid-1990s, inpatient margins began to improve, with aggregate inpatient margins being higher for urban than for rural hospitals. In 1997, urban hospital inpatient margins reached a peak of 18.0 percent, while the margins for rural hospitals reached a peak of 10.3 percent. Thereafter, inpatient margins began to decline: by 1999, urban inpatient margins had fallen to 13.5 percent and rural margins to 4.1 percent (see Table 5-1). Indeed, by 1999 over a third of all rural hospitals had negative Medicare inpatient margins (MedPAC, 2001).

During the late 1990s, the overall Medicare margin (including inpatient, outpatient, home health, skilled nursing, and psychiatric and rehabilitation

---

[3] The inpatient margin is calculated (in percentage terms) as the difference between inpatient payments and Medicare-allowable costs divided by inpatient payments (MedPAC, 2001). The same general approach is used for the overall Medicare margin and the total margin.

TABLE 5-1 Medicare Inpatient Hospital Margins, by Urban and Rural Location, 1990–1999

Year	1990	1991	1992	1993	1994	1995	1996	1997	1998	1999
Urban	−1.2	−2.2	−0.8	1.6	6.4	11.8	16.8	18.0	14.8	13.5
Rural	−3.7	−3.7	−1.4	−0.5	0.6	6.1	10.3	9.5	5.5	4.1

SOURCE: MedPAC, 2001.

units) for rural hospitals was several points lower than the inpatient Medicare margin (see Table 5-2). By 1998, when some Balanced Budget Act payment policies went into effect, the overall Medicare margin for rural hospitals had dropped 6 percentage points to –2.1 percent. In subsequent years, the overall margin has remained at approximately this level: –2.9 percent in 1999, –2.4 percent in 2000, –1.9 percent in 2001, and –3.9 percent in 2002 (MedPAC, 2001, 2004b).

In December 2003, Congress passed the Medicare Modernization Act, which modified Medicare payment policies for rural providers. These changes, effective in 2004, are expected to create an environment of greater financial stability for rural hospitals. For all rural hospitals, excluding those converted to community access hospital status by fall 2003, MedPAC expects the overall Medicare margin in 2004 to be 2.3, several points higher than the actual overall Medicare margin in 2002 of –3.9 (see Table 5-3).

Issues concerning the adequacy of rural hospital payments will continue to be raised, however, and rural hospital finance needs to be reviewed peri-

TABLE 5-2 Medicare Inpatient (1996–1999) and Overall (1996–2002) Rural Hospital Margins

Year	1996	1997	1998	1999	2000	2001	2002
Rural hospital Medicare inpatient margin	10.3	9.5	5.5	4.1			
Rural hospital Medicare overall margin	5.0	4.1	−2.1	−2.9	−2.4	−1.9	−3.9

SOURCE: MedPAC, 2001, 2004b.

TABLE 5-3 Overall Medicare Margins for Rural and Urban Hospitals

Year	2002 (actual)	2004 (estimated)
Rural hospitals	−3.9	2.3
Urban hospitals	2.6	1.3

NOTE: The table includes data from all hospitals covered by Medicare's inpatient Prospective Payment System, except those hospitals converted to critical access hospital status by fall 2003 (about 850).
SOURCE: MedPAC, 2004a: Chart 7-18.

odically. This is the case not least because the more generous margins[4] provided by private-sector health insurers that have helped sustain rural hospitals may be reduced in an increasingly price-competitive environment.

Medicare and Medicaid Payments to Primary Care Physicians

Similar to the situation with hospitals, rural physicians (see Appendix C for an overview) rely more on Medicare and Medicaid payments than their urban counterparts. Data from the 2000–2001 Community Tracking Study Physician Survey conducted by the Center for Tracking Health System Change reveal that rural physicians receive 38 percent of their payments from Medicare, while urban physicians receive 34 percent (difference significant at $p = 0.01$); likewise, rural physicians receive 19 percent of their payments from Medicaid, while urban physicians receive 14 percent (difference significant at $p = 0.01$) (Personal communication, K. J. Mueller, June 23, 2004). Medicare is also important to physicians in rural areas because it is a price leader, with private insurers often using fee schedules based on the Medicare schedules (Ginsburg, 2002).

The annual uprating and the geographic weighting factors of Medicare

---

[4] For the period 1996–1999, overall margins were considerably higher than overall Medicare margins for rural hospitals. Total margins for rural hospitals were 7.1 percent (1996), 6.6 percent (1997), 4.7 percent (1998), and 4.7 percent (1999). Overall Medicare margins for rural hospitals were 5.0 percent (1996), 4.1 percent (1997), −2.1 percent (1998), and −2.9 percent (1999) (MedPAC, 2001).

physician fee schedules have been controversial over the past few years. Medicare physician fee schedules are uprated using a sustainable growth rate (SGR) formula. Because of changes to that formula mandated by the Balanced Budget Act of 1997, Medicare payments to physicians were cut by 5.4 percent in 2002. Following congressional intervention, another 4.6 percent cut for 2003 was replaced by a 1.6 percent increase. Further congressional intervention through the Medicare Modernization Act of 2003 replaced cuts in 2004 and 2005 with 1.5 percent increases. Without additional legislation, cuts are likely to resume in 2006. MedPAC believes that the SGR formula fails to account for changes in the cost of physician services and that policy makers should consider alternative methods (MedPAC, 2001).

The above discussion is relevant to all physicians. Of special interest to rural physicians are the geographic price indexes used to calculate physician fees across the country. Physician fees are derived from three elements: the cost of physician labor to deliver a service, the practice costs associated with delivering a physician service, and the cost of professional liability insurance. Each element should fully reflect geographic differences across 89 payment areas. In response to arguments that physician work should cost the same regardless of where it is carried out, the geographic variation in the physician labor cost element has been weakened. The impact of the geographic variation in this element was further weakened by the Medicare Modernization Act of 2003, which called for a study by the General Accountability Office (GAO) (formerly the General Accounting Office) to assess the validity of the geographic adjustment factors used for each element of the fee schedule (MMA Section 413(c)(1)).

Individual states and the District of Columbia determine Medicaid fees for primary care physicians. These fees are low and significantly lower than the equivalent Medicare fees (GAO, 2003b). Low Medicaid fees have meant that many primary care physicians are unwilling to accept new Medicaid patients. In a national 2001 survey, only 54 percent of primary care physicians reported accepting most or all new Medicaid patients (Zuckerman et al., 2004). However, in rural areas, independent primary care clinics (and hospital outpatient departments) can qualify for rural health clinic status. Rural health clinics receive special "reasonable" cost reimbursement from Medicaid, i.e., higher than the standard Medicaid fee rates. The Benefits Improvement and Protection Act of 2000, however, allows states to replace cost-based reimbursement with the new Prospective Payment System. The financial impact of this legislation on rural health clinics is not yet known.

Medicare and Medicaid Support for Rural Health Clinics and Community Health Centers

A part of primary care in rural areas is provided through rural health clinics and community health centers (see Appendix C for an overview). Rural health clinics are heavily dependent on Medicare and Medicaid funding, with these two sources accounting for about 55 percent of their total revenues. Commercial and private insurance accounts for about 30 percent of total revenues, while revenues from uninsured, private pay, and free/reduced-cost care patients account for 15 percent (Gale and Coburn, 2003).

The overall financial health of some rural health clinics has been poor according to a survey carried out at the University of Southern Maine (Gale and Coburn, 2003). Data from the survey showed that total average expenses for these facilities ($681,457) exceeded average revenues ($641,683) by $39,774. Among more than 300 rural health clinics for which data were available, about half wrote off 5 percent or more and about 10 percent wrote off 15 percent or more of their charges as free or reduced-cost care. Further, about 8 percent of visits represented free or reduced-cost care. This survey predates the impact of the Benefits Improvement and Protection Act of 2000, which, as noted, allowed states to replace cost-based reimbursement with the Prospective Payment System. The impact of this legislation on the aggregate financial status of rural health clinics is not yet known.

Since their inception, community health centers have been heavily reliant on a patchwork of sources of public funds. During the 1990s, Medicaid funding increased proportionally while Section 330 funding decreased proportionally (HRSA, 2002). Of the total 2,000 revenues of the 748 community health centers receiving Section 330 grants, 34 percent came from Medicaid, 6 percent from Medicare, 25 percent from Section 330 and other federal grants, 14 percent from nonfederal grants (state and local grants, foundations), 6 percent from patients, and 15 percent from other private and public payers (BPHC, 2002).

Rural Resources for Dental Care

For more than 40 years, dental care has been funded predominantly by private sources (OPHS, 2000). Of total national dental expenditures in 2002, 44.0 percent was paid as out-of-pocket payments and 49.5 percent through insurance benefits (Levit et al., 2004).

According to a 1997 Behavioral Risk Factors Surveillance System survey, dental insurance coverage is strongly correlated with family income

TABLE 5-4 Dental Insurance Rates for Various Levels
of Family Income

Family Income	Percentage with Dental Insurance
Less than $15,000	31.5
$15,000–$24,999	40.6
$25,000–$34,999	54.1
$35,000–$44,999	67.8
More than $50,000	74.9

SOURCE: 1997 Behavioral Risk Factors Surveillance System,
Centers for Disease Control and Prevention (NIH, 2002).

(NIH, 2002). For families with income in the range $15,000–$24,999, 41
percent had dental insurance, whereas for those with income in the range
$35,000–$44,999, 68 percent had dental insurance (see Table 5-4). Since
incomes of families in rural areas are below those of their urban counterparts, there is less disposable income in rural areas to pay for dental services
and less likelihood that rural families will have dental insurance. Thus, there
are fewer economic resources per population available for dental services in
rural than in urban areas. This differential partly explains the shortage of
dentists in rural areas.

Medicaid and Medicare Support for
Nursing Homes and Home Health Services

The largest single source of payment for skilled nursing care is Medicaid. Two of three nursing home residents have their care covered at least in
part by Medicaid (GAO, 2003c). Under Medicaid, states and territories set
their own nursing home payment rates. Despite the fiscal pressures being
experienced at the state level, GAO found in a review of 19 states that during fiscal years 1998 through 2004, nursing home payment rates remained
largely unchanged (GAO, 2003c). However, GAO did report that state officials were warning about the possibility of reduced nursing home payments
after fiscal year 2004. Further, industry-sponsored studies found that nursing home costs for Medicaid-covered residents exceeded Medicaid payment
rates by an average of $9.78 per resident day in 2000 and an average of
$11.55 per resident day in 2001 in the 37 states included in the study (BDO
Seidman, 2003).

Legislative and administrative steps were taken in the late 1990s to reduce Medicare expenditures on home health care. The Balanced Budget Act of 1997 refined eligibility standards and changed the payment system. In addition, the Secretary of Health and Human Services initiated a program to reduce fraudulent use of the benefit. Over the period 1996–2000, the number of Medicare home health beneficiaries fell from 3.5 to 2.5 million, and over the period 1998–2000, the number of Medicare-certified home health agencies fell from about 10,000 to about 7,000 (MedPAC, 2004b).

MedPAC recently reviewed the impact of these changes on the availability and financial stability of home health agencies (MedPAC, 2004b). Since 2000, the number of Medicare-certified home health agencies has stabilized at about 7,000. Further, most communities have a home health agency: 99 percent of Medicare beneficiaries live in areas served by at least one home health agency. The vast majority of Medicare beneficiaries have a choice of provider, with 97 percent of Medicare beneficiaries living in areas served by more than one agency. MedPAC found that in the aggregate, freestanding home health agencies, representing about 70 percent of the total number of agencies, were financially stable in 2001 and projected to be so in 2004. The actual Medicare margin in 2001 was 17.0 percent for rural agencies and 16.0 percent for urban. The projected Medicare margin for 2004 is 16.9 percent for rural agencies and 16.3 percent for urban. In contrast, hospital-based agencies, representing about 30 percent of the total number of agencies, had an actual aggregate margin of 2.5 percent in 2001. The MedPAC report does not provide an analysis of the reasons for this wide divergence in aggregate margins between freestanding and hospital-based agencies. The lower margins impact rural areas more than urban since a greater proportion of hospital-based agencies are rural (48 percent) as compared with the rural proportion of freestanding agencies (35 percent) (MedPAC, 2004b). Lingering concerns about low Medicare home health margins in rural areas led to a recommendation in an earlier MedPAC report that Congress extend for 1 year 5 percent add-on payments for home health services provided to rural Medicare beneficiaries (MedPAC, 2003). This extension, effective April 2004, was included in the Medicare Modernization Act of 2003.

A 2000 survey carried out at the University of Minnesota examined the impact of closures of skilled nursing facilities and home health agencies attached to rural hospitals. The Balanced Budget Act of 1997 mandated use of the Prospective Payment System for skilled nursing care and home health services. The resulting reductions in payments led to the closure of some rural hospitals' post–acute care services. According to the results of the survey, 14 percent of hospitals that operated a skilled nursing facility in October 1997 had closed that facility by October 2000, and 13 percent of hospitals that operated a home health agency in October 1997 had closed that agency by October 2000 (Stensland and Moscovice, 2001).

These closures did not, however, lead to major reductions in access to care. In all but one case in which a hospital closed its skilled nursing facility, another such facility was operating within 15 miles of the hospital. Similarly, in all but one instance in which a home health agency was closed, another agency served the community (Stensland and Moscovice, 2001). It should be noted that the above survey was conducted before the Benefits Improvement and Protection Act of 2000 mandated higher payments for both skilled nursing facilities and home health services. Further, the Medicare Modernization Act of 2003 extended a 5 percent bonus payment for rural home health services through March 31, 2005. As a result, the current Medicare payment structure is more favorable than was the case when the above survey was carried out.

The Funding of Rural Emergency Medical Services

Rural emergency medical services (see Appendix C for an overview) rely heavily on volunteers. In addition, emergency medical services receive financial support mainly from transport fees and income from state and local taxes. A survey of 300 emergency medical services providers affiliated with critical access hospitals (83 percent response rate) revealed that on average, 62 percent of revenue was derived from transport fees (175 respondents) and 28 percent of revenue from state and local taxes (184 respondents) (Mohr, 2003).

Sources of reimbursement for transport fees include Medicare, Medicaid, commercial insurance or managed care, and private payers. Medicare is the largest source of these reimbursements. In 1998 on average, Medicare revenues accounted for 41 percent of providers' transport reimbursement fees for rural ambulance providers that bill Medicare (Mohr et al., 2000). This overstates the role of Medicare payments as many rural ambulance services do not bill for services. The national percentage of ambulance services that bill for services is not known. State-level data indicate considerable variation: some states report that very few of their rural service providers bill for services while others, such as Michigan and Wyoming, report that two-thirds to three-quarters of their rural service providers do so (Mohr, 2003).

According to state emergency medical service directors, a large proportion of rural emergency medical services are considered to be financially unstable (Knott, 2002). Further, in a recent report (see Box 5-1), GAO notes that the rural adjustment in the new ambulance fee schedule probably does not fully reflect the differences in the cost of providing ambulance services between rural and urban areas because the key factor affecting provider cost is annual trip volumes, which vary widely across rural counties (GAO, 2003a). The report recommends that CMS better target the Medicare rural payment adjustment for trips provided in rural counties with low population densities by adjusting base rates rather than the mileage rate (GAO, 2003a).

The above issues were addressed in the Medicare Modernization Act of 2003, which increased payment for trips of more than 50 miles, used a blended national and regional rate to set the fee schedule, and increased the base rate for ground ambulance services with low population densities. Looking to the future, the dependence of ambulance services on Medicare funding is likely to grow as the number of people aged 65 or over increases. In 1990, those aged 65 or over made up just 12 percent of the population but accounted for 36 percent of ambulance transports (Overton, 2002). Moreover, the cost of providing services may rise since some communities that have difficulties recruiting and retaining volunteer staff may have to hire paid staff (GAO, 2003a). On the other hand, an increasing number of rural volunteer providers are beginning to bill more aggressively for their services (GAO, 2003a). This is challenging for volunteer providers, particularly those who have no billing-related expertise.

Public Health Expenditures

Funding for public health comes from a wide array of sources, including local, state, and federal government programs; grants from foundations; reimbursements from insurance companies; and patient and regulatory fees. Recently published estimates based on National Health Account data show that over the period 1985–2000, public health spending increased from 1.05 to 1.32 percent of total health spending. During this same period, federal funds accounted for just under 30 percent of the total spent on public health (Frist, 2002).

Metropolitan and nonmetropolitan local public health agencies[5] have widely differing funding sources (NACCO, 2001) (see Table 5-5). In 1999, metropolitan local public health agencies received 58 percent of their funds

---

[5] It should be noted that focusing exclusively on local public health agencies for data on public health activities leaves out many rural communities without a local government public health infrastructure. There is currently no data source providing a comprehensive picture of all rural public health activities (Center for Rural Health Practice, 2004).

BOX 5-1
Ambulance Services: Medicare Payments
Can Be Better Targeted to Trips in Less Densely
Populated Rural Areas

In 2002, the Centers for Medicare and Medicaid Services implemented a new ambulance fee schedule, under which providers receive a base payment (dependent on the kind of services delivered) plus a mileage payment. There is a rural adjustment for the mileage payment, increasing payments for trips that begin in rural areas.

The General Accountability Office (GAO) found that trip volume is the key factor affecting differences in ambulance providers' cost per trip (GAO, 2003a). The majority of ambulance providers' costs reflect readiness—the need to have an ambulance and crew available. These costs are fixed. Thus, providers that make fewer trips tend to have higher costs per trip. In 2001, rural counties averaged 1,200 Medicare-covered trips (both emergency and nonemergency), while urban counties averaged 9,100 trips. Moreover, the number of Medicare-covered trips provided in rural areas varied greatly with population density. The quarter of rural counties that are most densely populated averaged 2,000 Medicare trips, while the quarter of rural counties that are least densely populated averaged just 300 Medicare trips.

Ambulance providers are paid on average 16 percent more for trips originating in the least densely populated quarter of rural counties than for trips originating in the most densely populated quarters of rural counties. This modest difference is much smaller than the nearly eightfold difference in average trip volumes (the key factor affecting cost per trip) between the least and most densely populated quarter of rural counties.

The GAO report recommends that the Centers for Medicare and Medicaid Services better target the Medicare rural payment adjustment for trips provided in rural counties with low population densities by adjusting base rates rather than the mileage rate.

from local government, 22 percent from state government (including federal pass-through funds), 14 percent from service reimbursement, and 3 percent directly from the federal government. By contrast, nonmetropolitan local public health agencies received 34 percent of their funds from local government, 35 percent from state government (including federal pass-through funds), 25 percent from service reimbursement, and 3 percent directly from the federal government.

The IOM's Committee on Assuring the Health of the Public in the 21st Century recently called for the Department of Health and Human Services to develop a comprehensive investment plan for a strong governmental public health infrastructure, with federal, state, and local governments providing adequate and sustainable funding for this purpose (IOM, 2003). Recent legislation—the Public Health Threats and Emergencies Act of 2000 and

TABLE 5-5 Sources of Funding for Local Public Health Agencies

	Metropolitan	Nonmetropolitan
Local public health agency	58 percent	34 percent
State government*	22 percent	35 percent
Service reimbursement	14 percent	25 percent
Federal government	3 percent	3 percent
Other	3 percent	3 percent

*Including federal pass through money.
SOURCE: NACCO, 2001.

the Public Health Security and Bioterrorism Preparedness and Response Act of 2002—aimed at improving bioterrorism preparedness will help strengthen the public health infrastructure.

Access to Capital for Rural Hospitals

Following the expression of concern (NACRHHS, 1999) about the need to repair or replace aging rural hospitals, the Walsh Center for Rural Health Analysis, University of Chicago, carried out a survey of 950 rural hospitals with under 50 beds to identify their capital needs and their ability to borrow funds (Stensland et al., 2002). As part of this survey, funded by the Health Resources and Services Administration, respondents were asked to estimate for their hospital the annual charges for borrowing $1 million. Of 221 respondents, 81 percent (178) were able to estimate their cost of capital, while the remainder (43) stated they would not qualify for a $1 million loan. The latter hospitals tended to be older, lower-volume facilities with operating losses. Likewise, a more recent survey, undertaken by the Rural Health Research Center, University of Minnesota, indicated that a significant proportion of critical access hospitals has difficulty raising capital. Of the critical access hospitals surveyed (95 percent response rate) 39 percent indicated that they had experienced an important capital need of at least $250,000 and had not tried to borrow the money because they had no chance of obtaining it (Gregg, 2004).

Two national programs have evolved over the years to help less credit-worthy hospitals—the Department of Housing and Urban Development's (HUD) Hospital Mortgage Insurance Program and the Department of Agriculture's Community Facilities Program. The Hospital Mortgage Insurance Program, commonly know as the HUD Section 242 Program, was established in 1968 to soften the impact of the sunsetting Hill-Burton Program. It has served primarily as a source of capital for urban facilities. The Community Facilities Program, started in 1972, is the lender of last resort to a wide range of eligible rural organizations in addition to hospitals. The two programs have provided only modest capital outlays to rural hospitals, only a quarter of which have been able to take advantage of them (Gregg et al., 2002). In addition to these two federal programs, there are about two dozen state-operated capital-related programs for which rural hospitals may be eligible. Almost three-quarters of these programs provide capital through grants, while a quarter do so through loans (Gregg et al., 2002).

Another, more limited program, focused on rural health care facilities, is the Southern Rural Access Program. This program is designed to help improve access to basic health care in eight of the most rural, medically underserved states in the country (Alabama, Arkansas, Georgia, Louisiana, Mississippi, South Carolina, (East) Texas, and West Virginia). To achieve these goals, the program emphasizes the development of rural health leadership, rural health networks, and revolving loan funds, as well as recruitment and retention of primary health care providers (Stewart et al., 2003). The program is funded by The Robert Wood Johnson Foundation and administered by the Pennsylvania State College of Medicine. As of November 2002, loans totaling $31 million[6] had been approved (Stewart et al., 2003).

One key to increasing access to capital for rural hospitals is to devise strategies for increasing their profitability. Recent survey data on critical access hospitals suggest that the longer hospitals operate in this capacity, the greater is the likelihood that they will be able to make investments that can have an impact on their continued financial profitability (Gregg, 2004). Implementation of the Medicare Modernization Act of 2003 can be expected to improve the operating margins of some rural hospitals. However, for those rural hospitals that are in serious financial difficulties and whose operations meet clear and pressing health care needs of their local populations, new policies are required.

---

[6] By the end of 2004, loans totaling $40 million are expected to have been approved (Personal communication, M. Beachler, June 2004).

Need for Financial Stability

Many parts of the rural health care delivery system have been financially fragile (for example, rural hospitals) or subject to payment uncertainties (for example, Medicare physician fees and Medicaid fees in general). In response, Congress has sought, most recently through the Medicare Modernization Act of 2003, to improve the financial climate for rural health care. Periodic reviews of the impact of this act on the financing of rural health care would, however, be prudent. Financial stability is required if rural health care facilities are to make the investments in human resource networks and information and communications technology required to deliver high-quality care on a consistent basis and establish a solid platform for the implementation of pay-for-performance systems.

THE FUNDING OF RURAL MENTAL HEALTH AND SUBSTANCE ABUSE SERVICES

In 1997, $85 billion, or 8 percent of total health care expenditures, was spent on mental health and substance abuse services. Of this amount, 86 percent ($73 billion) was for the treatment of mental health disorders and 14 percent ($12 billion) for the treatment of substance abuse disorders (Coffey et al., 2000). The majority of the funding of mental health and substance abuse treatment comes from public sources—the opposite of all health care spending. In 1997, public sources funded 58 percent of mental health and substance abuse treatment, as compared with 46 percent of all health services. The public sources were Medicaid (20 percent), Medicare (12 percent), other state and local sources (20 percent), and other federal sources (6 percent), while the private sources were private insurers (24 percent), out-of-pocket payments (16 percent), and other private sources (2 percent) (Coffey et al., 2000).

Private insurance, paying about a quarter of all mental health and substance abuse services, continues to place special limits on mental health benefits despite legislation designed to achieve parity between private mental health and general health insurance. The Mental Health Parity Act of 1996 prevented health plans from placing annual or lifetime financial limits on coverage of mental illnesses unless such limits existed for other medical services. Yet despite this federal legislation and state parity laws, the large majority of insured workers in employer-sponsored health plans in 2002 were still subject to special limits on mental health benefits: 74 percent of covered workers were subject to annual outpatient visit limits and 64 percent to annual inpatient day limits (Barry et al., 2003).

Mental health care services are provided in a variety of settings. As noted earlier, primary care physicians are important providers of mental health services in rural areas (DeGruy, 1996; Ivey et al., 1998). Mental health centers (formerly designated "community mental health centers" by the federal government) have shifted their focus to caring for those with serious and persistent mental illness and seriously emotionally disturbed children, largely because their block grant funding is restricted to these populations (Wagenfeld et al., 1994). Recently, the Bureau of Primary Health Care expanded the role of federally qualified health centers in providing mental health and substance abuse services for underserved populations (Lambert and Agger, 1995). Moreover, fewer rural than urban hospitals offer inpatient psychiatric services (Hartley et al., 1999). Overall, there are major shortages of mental health professionals in rural areas (see Appendix C). In September 1999, 87 percent of the 1,669 federally designated mental health professions shortage areas were rural counties (Bird et al., 2001).

Given the shortage of mental health and substance abuse services in rural areas, the committee believes a major assessment of the availability and funding of those services in rural areas is needed.

CONCLUSIONS AND RECOMMENDATIONS

Pay-for-Performance

The introduction of pay-for-performance approaches offers much potential to align payment incentives with the quality aims of the health system, but there is work to be done before these approaches can be implemented successfully in rural communities. Many rural providers lack the necessary quality infrastructure to participate in these payment programs. As discussed in Chapter 3, steps should be taken immediately to identify a set of standardized performance measures appropriate for use in rural communities, and technical assistance should be available to assist rural providers in establishing quality improvement programs. Chapter 6 addresses the need to invest in electronic health record systems that give clinicians immediate access to complete patient information and clinical knowledge, and provide the data needed to measure and continuously improve performance. It would also be wise to conduct demonstration projects in rural communities to test alternative approaches to pay-for-performance.

Recommendation 5. The Centers for Medicare and Medicaid Services should establish 5-year pay-for-performance demonstration projects in five rural communities starting in fiscal year 2006. During the first 18 months, the communities should receive grants and technical assistance for establishing processes to capture the patient data and other information needed to assess performance using a standardized performance measure set appropriate for rural communities. For the remaining 3.5 years, different approaches to implementing pay for performance should be tested in the various demonstration sites. The selected communities should be diverse with respect to sociodemographic variables, as well as the degree and type of formal integration of local and regional providers.

The Funding of Rural Health Care

Many rural health care delivery systems are financially unstable. Although significant steps have been taken to correct historical underpayment of rural providers under Medicare, the operating margins of many hospitals are still very low, and concerns about the equity of physician payments persist. Rural providers have been heavily impacted as states have modified eligibility criteria or lowered provider payments under Medicaid and the Children's Health Insurance Program in response to worsening state financial conditions.

Rural health care delivery systems must be financially stable if they are to finance investments in human resource networks and information and communications technology and to implement pay-for-performance initiatives. The committee concludes that an assessment is needed of the aggregate impact of changes in the Medicare program, state Medicaid programs, private health plans, and insurance coverage on the financial stability of rural health care providers, and that the Agency for Healthcare Research and Quality is well positioned to coordinate this assessment.

Recommendation 6. Rural health care delivery systems must be sufficiently stable financially to underwrite investments in human resources and information and communications technology and to implement pay-for-performance initiatives. The Agency for Healthcare Research and Quality should produce a report by no later than fiscal year 2006 analyzing the aggregate impact of changes in the Medicare program, state Medicaid programs, private health plans, and insurance coverage on the financial stability of rural health care providers. The report should detail specific actions that should be taken, if needed, to ensure sufficient financial stability for rural health care delivery systems to undertake the desired changes described in this report.

The Funding of Rural Mental Health and Substance Abuse Services

Given the shortages of mental health and substance abuse providers in rural areas, the committee concludes that a comprehensive assessment is needed of the availability of mental health and substance abuse services in rural areas (recognizing that another IOM committee is currently exploring the implications of the *Quality Chasm* report for the field of mental health and addictive disorders).

> **Recommendation 7. The Health Resources and Services Administration and the Substance Abuse and Mental Health Services Administration should conduct a comprehensive assessment of the availability and quality of mental health and substance abuse services in rural areas. This assessment should cover services provided in both primary care and specialty settings, and should include the following:**
>
> • **A review of (1) the various insurance and direct service programs in the public and private sectors that provide financial support for the delivery of mental health and substance abuse services and (2) the populations served by these payers and programs.**
> • **An evaluation of the adequacy of current funding and an analysis of alternative options for better aligning the various funding sources and programs to improve the accessibility and quality of these services. Attention should be focused on identifying and analyzing options designed to encourage collaboration between primary care and specialty settings.**

REFERENCES

Barry CL, Gabel JR, Frank RG, Hawkins S, Whitmore HH, Pickreign JD. 2003. Design of mental health benefits: Still unequal after all these years. *Health Affairs* 22(5):127–137.

BDO Seidman. 2003. *A Report on Shortfalls in Medicaid Funding for Nursing Home Care.* Washington, DC: American Health Care Association.

Bird DC, Dempsey P, Hartley D. 2001. *Addressing Mental Health Workforce Needs in Underserved Rural Areas: Accomplishments and Challenges.* Portland, ME: Edmund S. Muskie School of Public Service, Maine Rural Health Research Center.

BPHC (Bureau of Primary Health Care). 2002. *Uniform Data System National Rollup Calendar Year 2001 Data (Exhibit A: Total Revenue Received by BPHC Grantees).* [Online]. Available: http://www.bphc.hrsa.gov/uds/data.htm [accessed July 1, 2004].

Bridges to Excellence. 2003. *Rewarding Quality across the Health Care System.* [Online]. Available: http://www.bridgestoexcellence.org/bte/ [accessed April 28, 2004].

Center for Rural Health Practice. 2004. *Bridging the Health Divide: The Rural Public Health Research Agenda.* Bradford, PA: University of Pittsburgh, Center for Rural Health Practice.

Christensen DB, Holmes G, Fassett WE, Neil N, Andrilla CH, Smith DH, Andrews A, Bell EJ, Hansen RW, Shafer R, Stergachis A. 1999. Influence of a financial incentive on cognitive services: CARE project design/implementation. *Journal of the American Pharmacists Association* 39(5):629–639.

CMS (Centers for Medicare and Medicaid Services). 2004a. *National Voluntary Hospital Reporting Initiative.* [Online]. Available: http://www.cms.hhs.gov/quality/hospital/ [accessed April 29, 2004].

CMS. 2004b. *Premier Hospital Quality Incentive Demonstration Program.* [Online]. Available: http://www.cms.hhs.gov/quality/hospital/PremierFactSheet.pdf [accessed April 29, 2004].

Coffey RM, Mark T, King E, Harwood H, McKusick D, Genuardi J, Dilinardo J, Buck JA. 2000. *National Estimates of Expenditures for Mental Health and Substance Abuse Treatment.* Rockville, MD: Center for Substance Abuse Treatment and Center for Mental Health Services, Substance Abuse and Mental Health Services Administration.

Davidson SM, Manheim LM, Werner SM, Hohlen MM, Yudkowsky BK, Fleming GV. 1992. Prepayment with office-based physicians in publicly funded programs: Results from the children's Medicaid program. *Pediatrics* 89(4, Part 2):761–767.

DeGruy F. 1996. *Mental Health Care in the Primary Care Setting.* Washington, DC: National Academy Press.

Dudley RA, Frolich A, Robinowitz DL, Talavera JA, Broadhead P, Luft HS. 2004. *Strategies to Support Quality-based Purchasing: A Review of the Evidence (Technical Review No. 10). AHRQ Publication No. 04-0057.* Rockville, MD: Agency for Healthcare Research and Quality.

Fairbrother G, Siegel MJ, Friedman S, Kory PD, Butts GC. 2001. Impact of financial incentives on documented immunization rates in the inner city: Results of a randomized controlled trial. *Ambulatory Pediatrics* 1(4):206–212.

Frist B. 2002. Public health and national security: The critical role of increased federal support. *Health Affairs* 21(6):117–130.

Gale JA, Coburn AF. 2003. *The Characteristics and Roles of Rural Health Clinics in the United States: A Chartbook.* Portland, ME: Edmund S. Muskie School of Public Service, University of Southern Maine.

GAO (General Accounting Office). 2003a. *Ambulance Services: Medicare Payments Can Be Better Targeted to Trips in Less Densely Populated Rural Areas.* GAO-03-986. Washington, DC: GAO.

GAO. 2003b. *Medicaid and SCHIP: States Use Varying Approaches to Monitor Children's Access to Care.* GAO-03-222. Washington, DC: GAO.

GAO. 2003c. *Medicaid Nursing Home Payments: States' Payment Rates Largely Unaffected by Recent Fiscal Pressure.* GAO-04-143. Washington, DC: GAO.

Ginsburg PB. 2002. *Testimony before the Subcommittee on Health of the House Committee Ways and Means: Hearing on Physician Payments, February 28, 2002.* [Online]. Available: http://waysandmeans.house.gov/legacy/health/107cong/2-28-02/2-28gins.htm [accessed June 29, 2004].

Gregg W. 2004. *Best Practices in Obtaining Capital Funding for Major Hospital Projects: The Experience of CAHs.* San Diego, CA: Annual Meeting of National Rural Health Association.

Gregg W, Knott A, Moscovice I. 2002. *Rural Hospital Access to Capital: Issues and Recommendations.* Minneapolis, MN: Rural Health Research Center, University of Minnesota.

Hartley D, Bird D, Dempsey P. 1999. Rural Mental Health and Substance Abuse. In: Ricketts TC, ed. *Rural Health in the United States.* New York: Oxford University Press. Pp. 159–178.

Hibbard JH, Stockard J, Tusler M. 2003. Does publicizing hospital performance stimulate quality improvement efforts? *Health Affairs* 22(2):84–94.

Hickson GB, Altemeier WA, Perrin JM. 1987. Physician reimbursement by salary or fee-for-service: Effect on physician practice behavior in a randomized prospective study. *Pediatrics* 80(3):334–350.

Hillman AL, Ripley K, Goldfarb N, Nuamah I, Weiner J, Lusk E. 1998. Physician financial incentives and feedback: Failure to increase cancer screening in Medicaid managed care. *American Journal of Public Health* 88(11):1699–1701.

Hillman AL, Ripley K, Goldfarb N, Weiner J, Nuamah I, Lusk E. 1999. The use of physician financial incentives and feedback to improve pediatric preventive care in Medicaid managed care. *Pediatrics* 104(4, Part 1):931–935.

HRSA (Health Resources and Services Administration). 2002. *Experts with Experience: Community and Migrant Health Centers: Highlighting a Decade of Service (1990–2000).* [Online]. Available: ftp://ftp.hrsa.gov/bphc/pdf/chc/tenyear_report.pdf [accessed July 1, 2004].

IOM (Institute of Medicine). 2001. *Crossing the Quality Chasm: A New Health System for the 21st Century.* Washington, DC: National Academy Press.

IOM. 2003. *The Future of the Public's Health in the 21st Century.* Washington, DC: The National Academies Press.

Ivey SL, Scheffler R, Zazzali JL. 1998. Supply dynamics of the mental health workforce: Implications for health policy. *Milbank Quarterly* 76(1):25–28.

Knott A. 2002. *Access to Emergency Medical Services in Rural Areas: The Supporting Role of State EMS Agencies,* Minneapolis, MN: Rural Health Research Center, University of Minnesota.

Kouides RW, Bennett NM, Lewis B, Cappuccio JD, Barker WH, LaForce FM. 1998. Performance-based physician reimbursement and influenza immunization rates in the elderly: The primary care physicians of Monroe County. *American Journal of Preventive Medicine* 14(2):89–95.

Lambert D, Agger MS. 1995. Access of rural AFDC Medicaid beneficiaries to mental health services. *Health Care Financing Review* 17(1):133–145.

Levit K, Smith C, Cowan C, Sensenig A, Catlin A. 2004. Health spending rebound continues in 2002. *Health Affairs* 23(1):147–159.

MedPAC (Medicare Payment Advisory Commission). 2001. *Report to the Congress: Medicare in Rural America.* Washington, DC: MedPAC.

MedPAC. 2003. *Report to Congress: Medicare Payment Policy.* Washington, DC: MedPAC.

MedPAC. 2004a. *A Data Book: Healthcare Spending and the Medicare Program.* Washington, DC: MedPAC.

MedPAC. 2004b. *Report to Congress: Medicare Payment Policy.* Washington, DC: MedPAC.

Mohr PE. 2003. *Survey of Critical Access-Affiliated Emergency Medical Service Providers.* Bethesda, MD: Project HOPE Walsh Center for Rural Health Analysis.

Mohr PE, Cheng M, Mueller CD. 2000. *Findings from the 1999 National Survey of Ambulance Service Providers.* McLean, VA: American Ambulance Association.

Moscovice I, Davidson G. 2003. *Rural Hospitals: New Millennium and New Challenges.* Minneapolis, MN: Rural Health Research Center, University of Minnesota.

Mueller KJ, Stoner JA, Shambaugh-Miller MD, Lucas WO, Pol LG. 2003. Method for identifying places in rural America at risk of not being able to support adequate health services. *Journal of Rural Health* 19(4):450–460.

NACCO (National Association of City and County Health Officials). 2001. *Local Public Health Agency Infrastructure: A Chartbook.* Washington, DC: NACCO.

NACRHHS (National Advisory Committee on Rural Health and Human Services). 1999 (October 1). *Fiscal Year 2000 Recommendation: Rural Hospital Capital Need Loan Program.* [Online]. Available: http://ruralcommittee.hrsa.gov/recom_999.htm [accessed February 2004].

NIH (National Institutes of Health). 2002. *Oral Health U.S., 2002.* Bethesda, MD: National Institutes of Health, Centers for Disease Control and Prevention.

OPHS (Office of Public Health and Science, Office of the Surgeon General). 2000. *Oral Health in America: A Report of the Surgeon General.* Rockville, MD: National Institutes of Health, National Institute of Dental and Craniofacial Research.

Overton J. 2002. *Chapter 14: Reimbursement Trends in Prehospital Systems and Medical Oversight* (3rd Edition). Kuehl AE, ed. Dubuque, IA: Kendall/Hunt Publishing Company.

Premier, Inc. 2003. *Groundbreaking Medicare Project Underway with 278 Hospitals.* [Online]. Available: http://www.premierinc.com/frames/index.jsp?pagelocation=/all/informatics/qualitydemo/news/03-dec/280-hospitals.htm [accessed April 29, 2004].

Rewarding Results. 2002. *Aligning Incentives with High-Quality Health Care.* [Online]. Available: http://www.rwjf.org/publications/publicationsPdfs/cfp-rewarding_results.pdf [accessed April 28, 2004].

Rosenthal MB, Fernandopulle R, Song HR, Landon B. 2004. Paying for quality: Providers' incentives for quality improvement. *Health Affairs* 23(2):127–141.

Roski J, Jeddeloh R, An L, Lando H, Hannon P, Hall C, Zhu SH. 2003. The impact of financial incentives and patient registry on preventive care quality: Increasing provider adherence to evidence-based smoking cessation practice guidelines. *Preventive Medicine* 36(3):291–299.

Stensland J, Moscovice I. 2001. *Rural Hospitals' Ability to Finance Inpatient, Skilled Nursing and Home Health Care.* Minneapolis, MN: Rural Health Research Center, Division of Health Services Research and Policy, University of Minnesota.

Stensland J, Schoenman J, Mueller C, Singer A. 2002. *Capital Needs of Small Rural Hospitals: Final Report for the Office of Rural Health Policy.* Rockville, MD: Health Resources and Services Administration.

Stewart MK, Beachler M, Slayton D. 2003. Improving access to capital for health care infrastructure: The experience of the southern rural access program's revolving fund. *Journal of Rural Health* 19(Supplement):391–396.

Wagenfeld MO, Murray JD, Mohatt DF, DeBruyn JC. 1994. *Mental Health and Rural America: 1980–1993. An Overview and Annotated Bibliography.* ORHP, U.S. DHHS NIH Pub. No. 94-3500:1–116.

Zuckerman S, McFeeters J, Cunningham P, Nichols L. 2004. *Changes in Medicaid Physician Fees, 1998–2003: Implications for Physician Participation.* [Online]. Available: http://content.healthaffairs.org/cgi/content/full/hlthaff.w4.374/DC1 [accessed September 27, 2004].

6

Rural Health Care in the Digital Age[1]

SUMMARY

The health care sector is undergoing a critical transition from a delivery system aimed at providing episodic institutional care for the treatment of illnesses to an emphasis on information systems that support community-based care, with greater consumer involvement in the prevention and management of illness across the life span. The development of an information and communications technology (ICT) infrastructure is a critical element of this transition. ICT is a powerful tool with much potential to produce improvements in all six quality aims set forth in the Quality Chasm *report—safety, effectiveness, patient-centeredness, timeliness, efficiency, and equity—in all geographic areas. In rural America, appropriate use of ICT can bridge distances by providing more immediate access to clinical knowledge, specialized expertise, and services not readily available in sparsely populated areas. This chapter provides a discussion of the potential impact of ICT on health care delivery in rural areas; an overview of efforts under way to build local and national health*

---

[1] Much of this chapter was adapted from a commissioned paper by Thomas S. Nesbitt, Peter M. Yellowlees, Michael Hogarth, and Donald M. Hilty entitled "Rural Health in the Digital Age: The Role of Information and Telecommunicatioon Technologies in the Future of Rural Health" (March 18, 2004).

147

information infrastructures, with emphasis on developments in rural areas; and recommendations for addressing key issues and challenges specific to rural areas.

Over the past several decades, two important trends shaping health care delivery have accentuated the need for information and communications technology (ICT) as a key tool for supporting system improvement. First, there has been an exponential increase in medical knowledge. Sizable public and private investments in clinical research have led to a vastly expanded clinical knowledge base and many new drugs, medical devices, and other interventions, offering much potential to improve health and reduce pain and suffering. But translating new medical knowledge into practice has been difficult and slow (Balas et al., 1998).

It is no longer possible for an individual clinician, relying solely on the unaided human mind, to remain abreast of the expanding knowledge base and apply this knowledge appropriately to each patient (Becher and Chassin, 2001; Jerome et al., 2001). Computer-aided decision supports (e.g., reminders, prompts, and alerts) are needed to translate knowledge effectively into practice and safely utilize the many drugs and devices currently available.

Second, the life expectancy of the American public has been increasing (in part as a result of successes of the health care system), leading to an increased need for the management of chronic conditions (Anderson and Horvath, 2002; IOM, 2001a, 2003e; NCHC, 2002). About 40 percent of the American public have one or more chronic conditions, and approximately one-half of these individuals have two or more such conditions (Anderson and Horvath, 2002). Individuals with multiple chronic conditions see an average of six different clinicians per year and often receive care in multiple settings (e.g., hospital, rehabilitation facility, home health care provided in the community). Appropriate management of chronic conditions requires a high degree of communication among members of the care team and between clinicians and patients (as well as informal caregivers), and immediate access to complete patient records by all authorized users. Management of many chronic conditions also requires informed and engaged patients willing to modify health behaviors, monitor key health indicators, and implement complex medication and treatment regimens.

In the current health care delivery system, however, most critical patient information is recorded in handwritten medical records dispersed across various settings, including ambulatory practices, hospitals, nursing homes, and others. Clinical information does not travel with the patient, nor is it readily accessible by clinicians or the patient. Lacking computerized patient data, the current health system makes only minimal use of computer-based decision support tools (e.g., practice guidelines, preventive service reminders, potential drug–drug interaction alerts) to assist clinicians and patients in applying knowledge safely and effectively. For the most part, communication between clinicians and patients is limited to face-to-face visits or telephone calls, with only minimal use of e-mail.

Information technology is a particularly valuable tool for the redesign of the health care delivery system in rural areas. Compared with their urban counterparts, rural providers often practice on a much smaller scale and in greater isolation than urban providers; they tend to be generalists, but are often called upon to provide specialist services not available locally (Hart et al., 2002; Rosenblatt, 2000); and they must coordinate a larger number of transfers to facilities in distant locations (Melzner et al., 1997).

Improving the quality of health care ultimately requires improving the availability of health care information. The better information health care professionals have, the better they can diagnose illness, identify health improvement opportunities, discuss treatment options with patients, implement interventions, and achieve the desired outcomes (James, 2003). Similarly, information is necessary for patients to make choices consistent with their values and preferences. Finally, access to de-identified patient data can enhance health services research and population health surveillance systems. Central to this process is the need to maintain an electronic health record (EHR) that is complete and readily accessible to all providers and others with a need and right to know.

Computerized patient data and a secure network for communication and information exchange open up many opportunities to deliver services over the electronic highway. These "telehealth" services[2] range from relatively simple to very complex ICT applications, including e-mail communication between clinicians and patients; remote language and cultural interpreting; telemedicine (the provision of medical care from a distance using telecommunications technology); remote monitoring of patients in homes, intensive care units, or other locations; and eventually robotic surgery (Allen et al., 1997; Eadie et al., 2003; Field and Grigsby, 2002; Glick and Moore, 2001; Quintero et al., 2002).

---

[2] Telehealth is a broad set of applications using communications technologies to support long-distance clinical care, consumer and professional health-related education, public health, health administration, research, and EHRs (Matherlee, 2001).

Although an ICT infrastructure is a prerequisite to moving to a health system that employs telehealth care delivery and decision support, accomplishing these objectives involves more than the simple use of technology. It also involves major redesign of care processes, along with changes in the roles and relationships of clinicians and patients. In addition, developing the ICT infrastructure requires a community-based approach that leverages public and private resources across sectors. Thus making a successful transition necessitates careful attention to human, organizational, and technological factors (Castelnuovo et al., 2001; Stanberry, 2000; Yellowlees, 1997).

The next section of this chapter provides an overview of the many applications of ICT in rural health care environments to improve quality of care. The following two sections are devoted, respectively, to a discussion of the current status of ICT in health care and the identification of actions that can be taken to accelerate the adoption of ICT in rural settings. The final section presents conclusions and recommendations.

ICT APPLICATIONS IN RURAL SETTINGS

The development of an ICT infrastructure opens up many opportunities to improve health and health care in rural areas. Changes in health care delivery at all levels will result (BCG, 2003; Liederman and Morefield, 2003), including:

- Care at home and in the community
- Care provided in health care settings
  —Ambulatory and clinic care
  —Hospital care
- Population health

As important as the many new applications at each of these levels is the expected change in the distribution of care across levels. With the advent of telehealth, much care in the future will likely be provided in the patient's home. As discussed in Appendix C, the role of hospitals in many rural areas has already begun to change quite significantly in the last decade or two—from acute inpatient facilities to community health systems that encompass a good deal of ambulatory as well as inpatient care.

Following is a brief discussion of the ways in which care delivery in rural areas will likely change over the coming decade. For the most part, these changes are already under way in some geographic areas, and when available, examples and evidence of their impact are cited. Nonetheless, a great deal is still unknown about the benefits, costs, and intended and unintended consequences of the dramatic changes in care delivery that are unfolding.

Applications at Home and in the Community

ICT offers many new opportunities for rural residents to access health information, communicate with the health system from home for clinical and administrative purposes, and manage their chronic conditions more effectively. Likewise, rural individuals residing in community-based long-term care and assisted living facilities and the providers who care for them can greatly benefit from the ICT applications that will enable them to better coordinate care and health information across settings.

Enabling Access to Health Information

The Internet has enabled instant access to health information and resources on the Web, including medical journals, clinical guidelines, and databases encompassing the world's knowledge about conditions and diseases, as well as specially crafted patient-oriented materials, decision support tools, and online communities where patients can interact. However, the quality of information available on the Internet is highly variable (Berendt et al., 2001; Griffiths and Christensen, 2000). There are reliable sites that screen information carefully and organize the content to best meet the needs of consumers; examples are the National Library of Medicine's MedlinePlus and the Mayo Clinic website (NLM, 2004a; Mayo Clinic, 2004). Through partnerships between information providers and health care professionals, patients can be directed to quality sites by means of "information prescriptions" that can be filled at home for those with computer connections or at local public libraries (ACP, 2003; CIT, 2004). It is important to keep in mind that, as discussed earlier, low levels of health literacy and math skills in the U.S. population make communicating health information challenging. Indeed, an estimated one-half of the population likely experience difficulty understanding most health-related materials (IOM, 2004).

Communicating with the Health System

As patient and provider access to the Internet has grown, signs of a shift from face-to-face and telephone communication to e-mail and other

Internet-based communication modes are beginning to emerge, but this shift is very slow. Some rural health care providers have established Internet-based scheduling systems, such as the High Plains Rural Health Network (Versweyveld, 2001), that allow patients to schedule appointments in real time. The Geisinger Health System in Pennsylvania allows patient and their families to access their medical records to make appointments, check laboratory results, and order prescription refills (Rundle, 2002). In some instances, patients are also communicating with clinicians by e-mail.

Currently, most long-term care and assisted living facilities are limited in their technology capabilities, including administrative applications to process reimbursement claims and links to federal databases that monitor and track compliance with Medicare regulatory requirements, quality measures, and patient outcomes (IOM, 2001b). These facilities are now looking to implement ICT (i.e., EHRs and telemedicine systems) that can facilitate care coordination and management of health information as the patient moves through the care continuum (e.g., acute, hospital, assisted/long-term) or consults with physicians located in urban areas. ICT systems not only better support each "physician/facility handoff" by having the patient's documents and records available electronically through a single secure portal rather than distributed widely into different records for each provider, but also extend the facilities' reach to specialists and experts that are not available in rural areas, such as oncologists or neurologists.

Managing Chronic Conditions

Many ICT applications are designed to improve the management of chronic conditions, and these applications are increasingly being bundled into comprehensive chronic care management programs. Disease registries— online databases for monitoring certain chronic conditions—represent a low-cost method for online patient and provider data entry and monitoring of patient self-care. These registries include evidence-based guidelines, measures for improvement, and patient notifications for follow-up care. Numerous Internet sites provide condition-specific educational materials. The Internet also affords access to support groups (Fox and Fallows, 2003). Personal health records (PHRs) frequently include personalized education and health behavior monitoring tools (Waegemann, 2002).

As discussed in earlier chapters, rural areas often lack a critical mass of people with a particular chronic condition, making it difficult to form a support group, but there are now online support groups available for nearly every chronic condition. Online support groups, or chat rooms, may or may not be supervised by a medical care provider or "expert in that area of expertise" (White and Dorman, 2001), and little research has been conducted on the benefit of either sponsored or unsponsored electronic support (Johnson et al., 2001).

There are many examples of ICT applications, such as remote monitoring and telemedicine, being used for the home care of patients with chronic diseases including diabetes, asthma, and heart disease, as well as patients with chronic wounds, or mental health conditions (Kobb et al., 2003; Kobza and Scheurich, 2000; Romano et al., 2001; Smith et al., 2002). Remote monitoring integrates a variety of devices, including medication organizers and reminders, and devices that measure glucose levels, heart rate, blood pressure, weight, temperature, prothrombin time, and pulmonary function. Video-based telemedicine conferencing technologies for rural pediatric asthma patients has resulted in significantly reduced frequency of symptom experience and increased quality of life for both patients and their caregivers (Romano et al., 2001). Telemedicine has been shown to be effective in teaching behavioral self-regulation techniques to patients with chronic pain (Appel et al., 2002). In a study of elderly patients with congestive heart failure, in-person monitoring was found to be more effective in identifying edema and wheezing, but telemedicine yielded earlier identification of abnormal changes in nail color (Jenkins and White, 2001). Internet-based applications and telemedicine videoconferencing are increasingly being used for cognitive behavioral therapy and patient education for patients with disorders such as depression, anxiety, and substance abuse. Also, technology for therapy sessions is a growing resource for those needing long-distance care (Baigent et al., 1997; Hilty et al., 2003). Despite the promise of ICT, however, fewer than 200 home health programs are currently using these technologies, and only a very small portion of these programs are located in rural areas (Chetney, 2002; Field and Grigsby, 2002; Johnston et al., 2000; Smith et al., 2002).

Applications in Health Care Settings

ICT will likely have a very significant impact on providers in health care settings. Following is a brief discussion of applications in the areas of e-encounters, remote language and cultural interpretation, knowledge and decision support, storage and retrieval of diagnostic and health information, distance consultations and patient monitoring, and emergency care.

E-encounters

Estimates of physicians' use of e-mail to communicate with patients range from fewer than 10 percent of physicians to 25 percent (Bennett, 2002; Von Knoop et al., 2003). The slow adoption rate of e-encounters is likely attributable to the failure of most third-party payers to compensate providers for time spent in this manner (ACP, 2003). Some payers have begun to reimburse for e-mail consultations, however. For example, Blue Cross/Blue Shield of Massachusetts now pays physicians $19 for responding to patient e-mails, with about a $5 patient copayment. E-mail often takes the place of phone calls and brief office visits for such purposes as refills and adjustment of medications for both acute and chronic disease.

Remote Language and Cultural Interpretation

Providing professional language and cultural interpreting services presents a significant problem for rural providers, particularly in small clinics that serve patients from diverse ethnic and cultural backgrounds who may speak several different languages. Telecommunications technology has been used to address language barriers through the use of voice-only services that are available through a number of commercial telecommunications companies. Likewise, video has been used to deliver sign language interpretation to hearing- and speech-impaired populations in the United States, Sweden, and Australia (IOM, 2002b).

Knowledge and Decision Support

It is not unusual for each outpatient visit to generate at least one clinical question the physician is unable to answer (Bodenheimer et al., 2002). Only 30 percent of knowledge-based information needs perceived by internists during an outpatient visit are met (Covell et al., 1985). Thus there is a clear need for relevant medical knowledge at the point of care. This is especially true in rural areas, which rely extensively on generalists to handle a broad range of conditions. The impact of information interventions on the quality of care has been described in the literature (King, 1987; Klein et al., 1994; Lindberg et al., 1993; Marshall, 1992), with one study focusing specifically on the impact of a virtual library in rural areas (Richwine and McGowan, 2001). The potential role of medical librarians in reducing medical errors has also been documented (Homan, 2002).

In recent years, some progress has been made in enhancing rural providers' access to clinical knowledge. A number of mainstream medical publishers offer their content in web-enabled form, which dramatically facilitates distributed computerized access. University and community-based health systems also offer online, shared medical libraries that provide access to patient management tools such as clinical guidelines and condition-specific information and medical journals, in addition to links to information sources such as those offered by the National Library of Medicine and commercial sites. The National Library of Medicine provides grant funds for the development and integration of context-appropriate information, standards-based information management, and digital libraries; an example is the University of Iowa Hospitals and Clinics digital health sciences libraries, which provide information to physicians in six rural communities (D'Alessandro et al., 1988). Projects that involve rural public librarians and medical librarians bring quality health information and expertise to rural areas, with the goal of enabling health professionals to make more evidence-based decisions about their patient care practices and allowing the public to make informed decisions about their health. Much of this work is coordinated through the more than 4,800 medical libraries that are members of the National Network of Libraries of Medicine. This network works with a variety of intermediaries, including health care providers, population health professionals, public librarians, educators, community organizations, health advocacy groups, faith-based organizations, and self-help groups (NLM, 2004b). Network members have engaged in a number of projects funded by the National Library of Medicine and others related to the use of information technology in rural areas, including special projects for American Indian and Alaska Native communities (Duesing, 2002; Guard et al., 2000; McCloskey, 2000; McGowan, 2000; Pifalo, 2000; Spatz, 2000; Wood et al., 2003).

Decision support systems have also been shown to be highly effective and are expanding rapidly in use (Tierney, 2001). These systems consist of a knowledge database that links to clinical applications, such as alerts and reminders or evidence-based guidelines to help clinicians make decisions about patient care, and should make clinical practice safer, more accountable, and of higher quality. Decision support systems have been used in many settings, from primary care to the intensive care unit (Varon and Marik, 2002), and are increasingly available on the Internet in combination with systems for electronic prescribing and storage of EHRs (Smithline and Christenson, 2001). Something as simple and easy to use as a personal digital assistant can download several clinical application programs (e.g., drug interaction checking) to improve provider decision support immediately and inexpensively. Decision support systems designed to assist informal caregivers should be developed as well and are part of the promise for the future.

Storage and Retrieval of Diagnostic and Health Information

Store-and-forward applications are the methods by which still-frame images, voice or sound recordings, and medical data such as patient history, physical examination findings, and test results are captured, stored, and transmitted by e-mail or Internet posting. Alaska's telemedicine network, for example, uses store-and-forward e-mail protocols to transmit electrocardiograms to cardiologists in regional centers (Patricoski and Ferguson, 2003). Protocols have also been developed for teleneurology diagnostics in developing areas where real-time transmission of electroencephalogram data would be difficult (Patterson et al., 2001). Store-and-forward imaging applications are particularly effective in dermatology and ophthalmology. A number of studies have proven the clinical and cost effectiveness of these programs for screening and disease monitoring for retinopathy in diabetes and for melanomas and other skin cancers (Cummings et al., 2001; Liesenfeld et al., 2000; Rotvold et al., 2003). New systems that digitally capture and store radiology images (e.g., picture archiving and communication systems) eliminate the need for local film processing and reading.

Distance Consultations and Patient Monitoring

Real-time two-way video-based telemedicine entails a videoconference between a provider and a patient in a remote location with or without the referring provider being present. Teleconsultations can thereby bring the medical expertise of a specialist to the point of care. Many such programs entail attaching scopes to a two-way videoconferencing unit, such as a high-resolution, magnifying camera for observing dermatologic lesions or wounds, video otoscope, or video nasopharyngoscope. Electronic stethoscopes have been used for the transmission of audio output to pulmonologists and cardiologists. The interactive consultation also serves as a learning experience for the primary care provider. Generalists can have ready access to a broad array of specialists (e.g., radiologists, trauma surgeons) to assist with diagnosis and treatment, compensating for the specialist supply shortage. In addition, physicians can learn new surgical procedures (e.g., minimally invasive laparoscopic surgery) with a telementor and expert guide.

Telepsychiatry has been used quite extensively to increase access to psychiatric experts in areas with shortages of these specialists (which, as noted earlier, are common in rural areas (Armstrong and Frueh, 2002; Hilty et al., 2003; Jennett et al., 2003; Kennedy and Yellowlees, 2000; McLaren et al., 2003; Nelson et al., 2003; Nesbitt and Marcin, 2002). Software that uses the technique of cognitive behavioral psychotherapy has been shown to be reasonably effective for the treatment of simple depression, panic disorders, and simple phobias.

The use of telemedicine in inpatient settings will allow rural hospitals to keep more patients in the community and to raise the quality of care provided. For example, intensive care unit patients in rural hospitals can benefit from monitoring by intensivists located in urban areas through the use of videoconferencing and remote monitoring, resulting in reduced mortality, morbidity, and costs (Breslow, 2000; Celi et al., 2001; Marcin et al., 2004; Rosenfeld et al., 2000).

Emergency Care

Distance applications have become important to improving the quality of emergency care in rural areas. Several mechanisms now exist for wireless communication, including cordless, cellular, satellite, paging, and private mobile radio systems (Casal et al., 2004). These technologies, along with live video teleconsultations, are being employed for early-intervention, prehospital emergency care during ambulance transport. For example, studies of cardiac emergencies have shown that data transfer capabilities allow physicians to monitor electrocardiograms during prehospital care and determine whether and when to administer thromobolysis, saving valuable time in the critical moments of care by first responders (Keeling et al., 2003). Telemedicine is also being used for prehospital care related to abdominal sonography (Strode et al., 2003). One study forecasts a 15 percent decline in ambulance transports if prehospital telemedicine were used (Haskins et al., 2002).

As with care generally, telemedicine can play a significant role in emergency care in rural areas, bringing some of the expertise that may not be available locally into the emergency department via video consultation. A number of specialties have been incorporated into remote emergency rooms in this manner—initially radiology, then as technology advanced, cardiology, orthopedics, and surgery (Hashimoto et al., 2001; LaMonte et al., 2003; Lee et al., 1998; Levine and Gorman, 1999; Raikin et al., 1999; Sable, 2001;

Trippi et al., 1996). A North Carolina study found that use of teleradiology for diagnosis and treatment resulted in changes in nearly 30 percent of cases, as well as high levels of user satisfaction and confidence in these technologies (Lee et al., 1998). Another study in Vermont demonstrated significant benefit when trauma surgeons were available to rural emergency departments via videoconferencing during the initial evaluation and treatment of trauma victims (Ricci et al., 2003). ICT applications for ancillary services associated with emergency care, such as pharmacy, also are important to providers in rural areas. The value of these technologies for making more intelligent triage decisions has been established as well.

Population Health Applications

The systems and entities that protect and promote the population's health face a new set of challenges in the twenty-first century—obesity, toxic environments, a large uninsured population, and emerging threats such as antimicrobial resistance and bioterrorism (IOM, 2003b). The social, cultural, and global contexts of population health are also undergoing dramatic change. Genomics and informatics are extending the limits of human knowledge more rapidly than can be absorbed and acted upon. People, products, and germs can migrate more rapidly, and the nation's demographics are shifting in ways that will further challenge public and private resources (IOM, 2003b). While many population health surveillance systems are still operational, the need for next-generation technology is widely recognized. Advanced information technology systems are critical to the ability of population health systems to meet the new challenges to population health and preparedness.

Population health services and interventions are highly dependent on quality information to both locate and identify intervention targets, and then measure the effectiveness of the interventions. There is a need for intelligent information systems that enable population health data to be collected as a byproduct of care without adding to practitioners' workloads, and that allow for the use of more sophisticated data mining and analysis tools to interpret the increasing amounts of new data being collected (Mueller et al., 2003).

The Robert Wood Johnson Foundation is supporting the project Turning Point: Collaborating for a New Century of Public Health Initiatives to transform the population health system into a model that is more effective, more community-based, and more collaborative. Areas in which ICT could help population health officials perform their activities better include disease mapping and surveillance, quality of service, patient tracking for hospitals and clinics, services available within the community, vital statistics, environmental health, data analysis, information dissemination and health education, immunization, and laboratory reports (Burke and Evans, 2003). Improving ICT for the population health system would also allow rural areas to access the expertise of essential population health professionals at the state department of health as needed, making access to this specialized knowledge economically feasible for communities whose need for such services may be sporadic and immediate (NACRHHS, 2000). The use of ICT for communication among population health entities is essential as well for emergency preparedness, first-responder capabilities, and linkage to the Centers for Disease Control and Prevention's new Health Alert Networks (PHPPO, 2002). In addition, the National Library of Medicine has coordinated a project entitled Partners in Information Access for the Public Health Workforce, whose goals include organizing and delivering population health resources so they are easier to find and use (NLM Fact Sheet, July 2004: http://www.nlm.nih.gov/nno/partners.html).

CURRENT STATUS OF ICT IN HEALTH CARE

Several IOM committees and other expert groups have called for increased use of ICT in health care for quite some time. As early as 1991, the IOM recommended that the health sector transition from paper-based to computer-based patient records within 10 years (IOM, 1997). In 2000, the IOM Committee on the Quality of Health Care in America concluded that ICT "must play a central role in the redesign of the health care system" to achieve a significant improvement in quality (IOM, 2001a, p. 16). Numerous government panels, including the National Committee on Vital and Health Statistics (2001) and the President's Information Technology Advisory Committee (2001) have called for the development of a National Health Information Infrastructure (NHII). The Connecting for Health initiative of the Markle Foundation has engaged hundreds of public- and private-sector stakeholders in collaborative efforts to advance interconnectivity and the use of EHRs (Markle Foundation, 2003). Recently during his State of the Union address, President Bush announced a commitment to ensuring that all Americans have EHRs within 10 years (WH, 2004a).

Implementing these technologies requires the development of an ICT infrastructure with major building blocks that include the following:

- *National data standards*—specifications for the collection, coding, and exchange of clinical and other information pertaining to patients.
- *EHRs*—computer-based patient records maintained by health care providers (e.g., hospitals, ambulatory settings, nursing homes, home health providers) that include a spectrum of clinical and patient data, such as demographic data, diagnostic and treatment data, ancillary test results, progress notes, and insurance and billing data.
- *PHRs*—computer-based patient records maintained by patients and informal caregivers that include such information as preventive health information, health education material, medication and other treatment plans for chronic conditions, and tracking of health behaviors and key indicators.
- *Information exchange networks*—clinician and patient access to a secure environment on the Internet for communication and information-sharing purposes.

Establishing an ICT infrastructure for health care will require the participation of many stakeholders. The federal government, in collaboration with private-sector standards-setting bodies, must promulgate the data standards that will allow for the meaningful exchange of patient and other data. Providers must migrate from paper medical records to EHRs, and patients must obtain and use PHRs. Public–private partnerships must be created at the community level to establish and maintain information exchange networks. The partnerships necessary to build the networks must also expand beyond the health sector to other sectors in the local community, such as education and regional businesses that can benefit from improved ICT infrastructure.

The use of ICT is growing in rural areas. While the implementation of ICT is currently incomplete and uneven across the domains of the health sector in both urban and rural areas, overall, rural areas lag behind urban in establishing the critical ICT building blocks outlined above. This section provides an overview of the current status of ICT adoption in rural areas as background for further discussion on how to address barriers to the development of a more comprehensive rural health ICT system.

Internet Connections

With the advent of the Internet, access to health information has improved dramatically in the last decade (Anderson, 2001b; Nesbitt et al., 2002). As of 2003, about 63 percent of the U.S. adult population was using the Internet, and an estimated 93 million of these 126 million people were using it to access health information (Madden and Raine, 2003). Nearly one-third of these users reported having broadband connections. One study found that 40 percent of all Internet users had sought advice or information about health or health care, and one-third stated that the information obtained had affected a health care decision (Helms, 2001). In a survey by the Pew Internet and American Life Project, 61 percent of respondents said the Internet had improved the way they took care of themselves either "a lot" or "some." And while some are concerned about the quality of online health information, the ability to contribute to a more informed patient population is embraced by many health professionals.

Although Internet access is growing, however, some groups lag behind, including racial and ethnic minorities, those with low incomes and educational levels, older people, and residents of rural areas (Madden and Raine, 2003). Progress is being made in closing some of these gaps. Between 1998 and 2001, for example, the growth of Internet use in rural areas increased from 24 to 53 percent (OTP, 2004). A community-based effort to build the necessary telecommunications infrastructure and provide training for computer literacy will help residents to improve information access and communication for multiple purposes, including health care.

The proportions of practicing physicians who work online from home, from their personal office areas, and from their clinical work areas are all increasing (Taylor and Leitman, 2001). A nationwide survey of 834 physicians comparing 1999 and 2001 data found that by 2001, 55 percent of all practicing physicians were using e-mail to communicate with professional colleagues and 34 percent to communicate with their support staff, while 42 percent of all physicians worked in practices with websites. However, only 13 percent of all doctors were communicating with any of their patients via e-mail, and 7 percent of physicians were not online anywhere (Taylor and Leitman, 2001). A survey of the approximately 60,000 members of the American Academy of Family Physicians (25 percent of whom practice in rural areas) found that 80 percent were connected to the Internet, and rapid migration to either digital subscriber line (DSL) or cable modems for high-speed networks was occurring (Kibee, 2004).

Electronic Health Records

Results of an industry survey conducted in 2002 indicate that just 13 percent of private-sector inpatient facilities and 14–28 percent of ambula-

TABLE 6-1 Electronic Data Capture by Regional Population

		Nonmetropolitan			Metropolitan	
	Total	< 25K	25–49.9K	< 250K	250K–1million	> 1 million
Mean	38.0%	29.6%	35.8%	35.4%	39.9%	41.7%
Median	25.0%	10.5%	21.0%	25.0%	30.0%	30.0%

SOURCE: Lorence et al., 2002.

tory care facilities use EHRs (Brailer, 2003). As shown in Table 6-1, EHR adoption in metropolitan areas is 1.5 times greater than in small rural areas (Lorence et al., 2002). As discussed below, factors that have contributed to the slow adoption of EHRs in the health care sector include the lack of national data standards and finance issues.

Several factors that have precipitated the lag in widespread adoption of EHRs (e.g., organizational leadership, financing, and technology infrastructure) are now being addressed and are discussed later in this chapter. To facilitate national adoption of EHR systems, the IOM built upon its original 1991 report on the computerized patient medical record and released its 2003 Letter Report on Key Functionalities of EHRs (http://www.nap.edu/catalog/10781.html?npi_ newsdoc073103). The report provides a list of the ICT applications associated with each functionality, as well as a plan for progressively implementing the applications over the next 8 years.

Personal Health Records

EHRs are also important because they are the foundation for a computerized PHR. PHRs allow individuals access to portions of their EHR (e.g., diagnoses, medications, laboratory test results) through a secure portal. Patients may enter information as well, such as diet, exercise, adherence to treatment plans, and over-the-counter medications. PHRs can include (1) offline records that can be carried in paper-based files/booklets or on a CD-ROM or smart card; (2) Web-based commercial PHRs, whereby one's health information is stored on a secure webpage; (3) functional/purpose-based PHRs, which are Web-based records related to a specific service, such as emergency care; (4) provider-based PHRs, whereby the provider or health plan makes some of the patient's health information available on the provider's website; and (5) partial PHRs, whereby patients keep a file of health information and literature about diseases and conditions downloaded from the Web, which can also be used by the Web provider for marketing purposes (Waegemann, 2002).

A recent review of 12 web-based PHRs, however, found that these systems had limited capabilities and were difficult to navigate (Kim and Johnson, 2002). Most PHRs are simply a file of data; few have decision support capabilities that would help patients manage their chronic conditions. Not surprisingly, then, only a small fraction of the population use PHRs (Waegemann, 2002). PHRs may ultimately prove to be a highly valuable tool to assist patients with their care; however, much work needs to be done to improve their functionality, usefulness, and appeal to consumers.

Telemedicine

As discussed earlier, telemedicine has a number of applications in patient care, education, research, administration, and population health (Wakefield, 2002) and has the potential to be an important means of equalizing the differential availability of resources in rural and urban areas (Hartley et al., 2002; Wholey et al., 2003). The federal government and some academic institutions have used two-way videoconferencing in health care for almost 40 years, but not on a widespread basis because of costs, provider reluctance, lack of perceived need, and limited telecommunications infrastructure (Perednia and Allen, 1995). With the introduction of digital telephone lines and the decreasing cost of hardware and software in the 1990s, videoconferencing is on the rise as a medium for providing health services (Hassol et al., 1997a,b). The Department of Commerce recently reviewed the telehealth projects supported by a number of federal agencies[3] and estimated that allocations of $332 million were made for such projects in 2001 (OTP, 2004). Because of the disjointedness of the projects, however, one of the key recommendations in the Department of Commerce report is the development of a national database for telehealth. The committee concurs

---

[3] U.S. Department of Agriculture, Department of Commerce, Department of Defense, Department of Education, Department of Energy, Department of Health and Human Services, Department of Justice, National Aeronautics and Space Administration, Veterans Administration, and Federal Communications Commission.

that greater coordination and a centralized database for monitoring federally sponsored telehealth programs would be beneficial.

Many rural communities and providers are actively engaged in telehealth. A 1997 survey of 2,472 nonfederal rural hospitals indicated that 30 percent (700) of rural health care organizations were engaged in some form of telehealth (OTP, 2004). A 1999 study by the Agency for Healthcare Research and Quality (AHRQ) identified 455 telemedicine projects worldwide, 362 of these in the United States, 120 of which were in rural areas. Patient volumes in these latter projects remain low given the demographics of rural areas. The AHRQ study found the most common applications to be consultations or second opinions (80 percent), diagnostic test interpretation (47 percent), chronic disease management (36 percent), posthospitalization or postoperative follow-up (28 percent), emergency room triage (26 percent), visits by a specialist (22 percent), and services in patients' homes (14 percent) (OTP, 2004). Many of the projects included more than one application.

Technical Requirements

ICT applications depend on the exchange of data among providers, patients, and vendors. For the most part, exchanging data requires access to digital lines, along with national data standards to facilitate meaningful communication and protect confidentiality.

For the majority of health care ICT applications, especially those involving the transmission of large amounts of information for real-time interaction, higher-bandwidth digital lines are required. Telemedicine for intensive care units using two-way interactive video, for example, requires high-speed digital lines with large bandwidth (e.g., fiber optics, DSL).[4] For some simpler applications, such as the transfer of still images using store-and-forward technology, a simple Internet service provider (ISP) connection over ordinary telephone lines may be adequate.

While the penetration of basic telephone service is at about 95 percent for rural households and essentially 100 percent for rural hospitals and clinics, access to higher-speed digital lines is limited. A study conducted in 2000 found that cable modem service and DSL were offered in fewer than 5 percent of towns with a population of 10,000 or less; by comparison, modem service is offered in more than 65 percent of cities with 250,000+ popula-

---

[4] Bandwidth is the maximum amount of data (measured in bits) that can travel a communications path in a given time (measured in seconds).

tion, and DSL is available in more than 56 percent of all cities with 100,000+ population (Allen, 2001). This aspect of the digital divide is one of the greatest challenges for rural telehealth, as well as other rural commerce.

As noted earlier, data standards[5] are another important aspect of ICT requirements. To be most user-friendly, information exchanges require common standards for how the data are packaged, how systems interact, and what vocabulary is used to represent the information (IOM, 1997). When the sending and receiving systems use the same data standards, health information can flow more easily from one system to another. Telehealth applications such as the transmission of radiological images, physician order entry systems, and home care medical device monitoring systems rely on data communication standards to speed transmission and improve connections among users (typically referred to as increasing interoperability and scalability). However, poor system interoperability, limited data comparability, and the need to improve data quality and integrity have been cited as major obstacles to the electronic exchange of health information in both urban and rural settings (Lumpkin, 2000). Currently, vendors of certain imaging technologies (e.g., teleradiology) have employed a common standard (DICOM) for packaging and transmitting images in their systems, while vendors of other applications are only now beginning to incorporate the federal government's recommended standards. Accelerating the promulgation of national data standards is one element of a comprehensive plan to facilitate the adoption of EHRs, and substantial progress has been made to this end, particularly in the past 3 years. The standards developed are international in scope and tied to the National Library of Medicine's Unified Medical Language System.

ACCELERATING THE ADOPTION OF ICT IN RURAL SETTINGS

Recent years have seen a great deal of momentum and some tangible progress toward the development of an NHII. The envisioned NHII has been defined as a set of technologies, standards, applications, systems, values, and laws that support all dimensions of the health system—personal health management, provider care delivery, population health, and research (NCVHS, 2001). More specifically, the NHII initiative is a cohesive and

---

[5] Data standards are methods, protocols, terminologies, and specifications for the collection, storage, and exchange of information.

comprehensive plan to design information networks comprising the following elements:

- Communications technologies such as high-speed telecommunications networks, computer-based systems, and wireless systems
- Data standards such as common standards for medical terminology, encoding and transmitting data, and formatting electronic documents
- Application programs for EHRs, telemedicine, and patient self-management
- Certain systems that relate to the underlying electronic architecture, databases for collecting and storing data, and medical knowledge sources
- Values and laws to ensure appropriate regulatory oversight, consumer protection, and government support for vulnerable populations

Building the NHII is an enormous undertaking that will likely take a decade or more to complete, but the process is well under way. A detailed discussion of the many ongoing efforts related to the establishment of the NHII can be found elsewhere (IOM, 2003d; Javitt, 2004). Following is a brief summary of recent developments in four key areas: federal leadership, patient privacy laws, data standards for connectivity, and finance.

Federal Leadership

In May 2004, the White House announced a new national initiative aimed at establishing the NHII and implementing EHRs over the next 10 years (WH, 2004c). One key component of this initiative was the establishment of the Office of the National Coordinator for Health Information Technology in the Department of Health and Human Services (DHHS) to facilitate higher levels of interagency strategic development and coordination. The National Coordinator serves as the chief architect and strategic planner for coordinating federal, state, and private-sector activities directed at establishment of the NHII. The National Coordinator was tasked with providing a comprehensive NHII implementation plan to the Secretary of DHHS by July 21, 2004, followed by delivery to the President (WH, 2004c).

Patient Privacy Laws

The Health Insurance Portability and Accountability Act of 1996 (HIPAA) set standards for administrative and financial transactions and the privacy and security of personal health information. The rules that emerged from the HIPAA regulations require that all health care providers, clearing-houses, and health plans implement these standards by the compliance date specified for each. The Administrative Simplification provisions identified data exchange standards and code sets for representing the information; compliance was required by October 16, 2003 (with the option of filing for a 1-year extension). The privacy rules establish the minimum standards required for the protection of information within an organization and among business associates, as well as stipulations for obtaining authorization for disclosure and de-identification of information. Compliance was required by April 14, 2003. The security standards govern the administrative procedures, physical safeguards, and technical security services and mechanisms for ensuring data protection using all media and for storing, maintaining, and exchanging information. These rules were just completed, and compliance is required by April 21, 2005.

Data Standards for Connectivity

In 2002, the Consolidated Health Informatics (CHI) initiative was established as part of the Office of Management and Budget's eGOV efforts to streamline and consolidate government programs among like sectors (OMB, 2000). The CHI, with input from the National Center on Vital and Health Statistics and various private-sector standards-setting bodies, identifies data standards for government-wide adoption. Acting on advice from CHI, in June 2003 the Secretary of DHHS assumed a lead role in the promulgation of data standards for key areas, including reporting of laboratory results, digital radiology reporting, medical device communications, pharmacy communications, and clinical data communications. A great deal of standards-setting work remains to be done, and a recent IOM report provides a roadmap for additional progress in this area (IOM, 2003d). Designation of the National Center on Vital and Health Statistics as the preeminent health information policy advisory group of the federal government, the development of its vision statement for the NHII, the CHI collaboration, and the recent promulgation of some data standards have established a policy process and generated a widespread expectation that the federal government will continue to address this important issue in a thoughtful, coordinated, and strategic manner.

Finance

Some modest first steps have been taken to assist providers and communities in investing in ICT. In fiscal year 2001, more than $30 million in federal grants was available to support Indian Health Service and Alaskan health care infrastructure initiatives, including telehealth technologies (IHS, 2000). In fiscal year 2004, Congress appropriated $50 million to help small and rural hospitals invest in ICT (AHRQ, 2003a). In fiscal year 2005, an additional $50 million will be made available to communities to plan and implement local/regional health information infrastructures (AHRQ, 2004b).

Although it is too early to assess the full impact of this and the other developments described above, building the NHII has clearly become an important national priority. Below the committee identifies actions that should be taken to ensure that rural areas have an opportunity to both contribute to and benefit fully from the NHII.

CONCLUSIONS AND RECOMMENDATIONS

Building the NHII over the coming decade presents both opportunities and challenges for rural communities. As discussed above, all communities stand to derive sizable benefits from the NHII, and these benefits may be even more substantial in rural communities, where the NHII has the potential to greatly enhance residents' access to providers and services. At the same time, however, rural communities are at risk of being left behind. Some are poorly prepared to participate in the information age, having little or no access to the Internet and populations with minimal ICT experience. Given their limited financial resources (see Chapter 5) and the small scale of rural provider organizations (see Appendix C), most rural health care systems will need financial and technical assistance to establish EHRs and secure platforms for data exchange.

Although there are challenges to be overcome, rural communities also have unique strengths to build upon and may represent excellent sites for community-based ICT demonstrations involving public- and private-sector partnerships. Rural health care systems are less complex than those in urban areas, and the scarcity of resources in rural settings provides strong incentives for collaboration among all stakeholders. Moreover, rural hospitals and nursing homes are far less likely than their urban counterparts to have made major investments in information systems in the past, so they do not confront the challenge of converting from these legacy systems to the NHII.

In this section, the committee lays out a strategy and recommendations for ensuring that no rural community is left behind as the nation builds the NHII, and that rural communities, like their urban counterparts, have the opportunity to adopt innovations if they choose to do so. This strategy consists of six action items: (1) including a rural focus in the NHII plan, (2) providing all rural communities with high-speed access to the Internet, (3) improving the consistency of regulatory and payment policies, (4) providing financial assistance to rural providers for investment in EHRs and ICT, (5) fostering ICT collaborations and demonstrations in rural areas, and (6) providing ongoing educational assistance to rural communities so they can make the best use of ICT.

A Rural Focus in the NHII Plan

With the establishment of the Office of the National Coordinator for Health Information Technology, the federal government has assumed a leadership role in the development of the NHII over the next 10 years. To achieve this goal, the NHII Coordinator must implement a comprehensive strategy, operational plan, and budget.

If rural communities are to participate fully in the NHII, it is essential that the national planning process take into consideration the specific challenges they confront and target program activities and resources to meet these challenges. The committee believes that the involvement of rural health leaders in the development of the NHII will be critical to its successful implementation in rural areas. The initiation of an ongoing dialogue between the National Coordinator and public- and private-sector rural health leaders would also likely result in the identification of numerous opportunities to coordinate ICT development with other rural health programs and to better leverage public- and private-sector investments.

The Office of Rural Health Policy (ORHP) in DHHS's Health Resources and Services Administration (HRSA) serves as a focal point for many rural health programs and activities at the national level. ORHP also provides administrative support for the DHHS Rural Task Force, established in 2002 by the Secretary of DHHS (ORHP, 2002). This task force of federal and state agencies involved in rural health projects is charged with streamlining and coordinating their initiatives for better overall strategic planning and development of rural health care delivery systems. With input from ORHP and the DHHS Rural Task Force, the NHII Coordinator would be better positioned to meet the needs of rural communities.

Recommendation 8. The Office of the National Coordinator for Health Information Technology should incorporate a rural focus, including frontier areas, into its planning and developmental activities for the NHII.

• The NHII strategic plan should include a component that is specific to rural and frontier areas, and this component should provide the programmatic and financial resources necessary for rural areas to participate fully in the NHII.
• The Office of Rural Health Policy should be designated as the lead agency for coordination of rural health input to the Office of the National Coordinator for Health Information Technology. In providing this input, the Office of Rural Health Policy should seek the expert advice of the Department of Health and Human Services' Rural Task Force.

High-Speed Access to the Internet

Many health-related ICT applications require access to high-speed Internet connections; however, broadband networks have not yet reached many rural communities (Wellever, 1999). Broadband networks can benefit rural communities as a whole by giving local firms direct access to customers, suppliers, and larger markets, thus making it less expensive and more efficient for firms to locate in rural areas (McMahon and Salant, 1999). In addition, these networks make it possible for residents of small towns to participate in distance education, training, and learning opportunities, a capability that is particularly important for building a health professions workforce and promoting health literacy (see Chapter 4). It is essential that a cross-sector, community-based approach serve as the foundation for developing high-speed networks in rural areas. This approach would result in coordination and collaboration across sectors, which could decrease costs and improve efficiencies related to ICT infrastructure development.

Efforts are under way to address this issue, but more needs to be done. In January 2003, the U.S. Department of Agriculture's Rural Utilities Service expanded funding of its rural telecommunications development efforts to more than $1.4 billion, allocated through its Rural Broadband Loan and Loan Guarantee Program (RUS, 2004). The Department of Commerce has also provided grants to rural areas to facilitate the completion of broadband networks; an example is the Northeast Wyoming Economic Development Coalition, which covers five counties (Mueller et al., 1999). In April 2004, the President announced the goal of making advanced broadband networks available and affordable to every American by 2007, including those in rural areas (WH, 2004b). The announcement emphasized the importance of partnerships among government agencies; regional commissions; state, local, and tribal governments; and industry. Some private vendors are now working with local communities to build lower-priced wireless broadband networks (Davidson, 2004). These networks use WiMax technologies that extend the wireless service radius to 30 miles, thus covering many rural areas. Additional resources should be made available as needed for the expansion of wired and wireless broadband networks to ensure that all rural communities have access to such networks by 2007. Where needed, programs should provide assistance for the internal wiring of health care provider facilities and for connection to the telecommunications infrastructure.

Rural areas face another barrier in use of the Internet—the cost associated with the use of telecommunications lines. Surcharges and administrative fees levied by local area telecommunications access (LATA) networks often make data exchange prohibitively expensive, and this is especially true when the data transmission is between geographic areas located in different LATA networks. LATA companies need to afford rural health providers a "safe harbor" from excessive surcharges and/or administrative fees.

The federal and state governments provide some financial assistance to certain rural providers for the cost of data transmission. State funds, collected from telecommunications service providers, are generally used to supplement the federal program (Haas, 2001). Reimbursement for line usage is available for rural providers through the Universal Service Administrative Company's Rural Health Support Mechanism (with oversight provided by the Federal Communications Commission as per the Telecommunications Act of 1996).[6] Yet of the $400 million in funds that has been authorized for this purpose under the Telecommunications Act, only 10 percent has been allocated because of a number of impediments (USAC, 2004). Eligibility for these funds is too limited,[7] and should be expanded to include all rural providers (e.g., nursing homes, hospices, home health care providers, substance abuse treatment centers, emergency service providers,

---

[6] The Fund provides discounts for telecommunications costs to rural health care facilities by subsidizing the difference between rural charges compared to those for metropolitan areas.

[7] Eligibility for Rural Health Support Mechanismis strictly limited to public or nonprofit organizations categorized as an academic health center, community/migrant health center, local health department, community mental health center, nonprofit hospital, rural health clinic, or consortia of the above.

and private for-profit providers), and be on equal footing with the Universal Service Administrative Company's E-rate Program for schools and libraries. Currently, participants in the Rural Health Support Mechanism receive reimbursement for 25 percent of ISP charges, whereas schools and libraries receive up to 90 percent. Lastly, the administrative paperwork associated with the program needs to be simplified significantly, and outreach and education about the program expanded to attract more participants. The committee supports a thorough review of the structure and function of the Rural Health Care Support Mechanism programs as a priority for strengthening the financial resources available to rural communities.

> **Recommendation 9. Congress should take appropriate steps to ensure that rural communities are able to access and use the Internet for the full range of health-related applications. Specifically, consideration should be given to:**
>
> • **Expanding and coordinating the efforts of federal agencies to extend broadband networks into rural areas.**
> • **Prohibiting local area telecommunications access networks from imposing surcharges for the transfer of health messages across regions.**
> • **Expanding the Universal Service Fund's Rural Health Care Program to allow the participation of all rural providers and to increase the amount of the subsidy.**

Consistent Regulatory and Payment Policies

The regulatory and payment environments have a significant impact on the ability of providers to make the best use of ICT. Currently, the use of telemedicine and other ICT applications is impeded by the absence of clear and consistent definitions and requirements across (1) state governments that license health professionals; (2) health care organizations (e.g., hospitals, health plans, nursing homes) that credential clinicians for practice within the organization; and (3) major payers, such as Medicare, that establish payment policies for telemedicine services.

Some programs define the telemedicine "site of care" as the location of the patient, while others use the location of the clinician. There is much variability in state licensure requirements, with some states prohibiting any form of telemedicine encounter unless the clinician possesses a license for the state in which the patient is located, and others allowing consultations but not "treating relationships" with clinicians. Similarly, there is variability in the credentialing policies of health care provider organizations, in part reflecting the requirements of accreditation programs such as those of the Joint Commission on Accreditation of Healthcare Organizations and the National Committee for Quality Assurance. Moreover, Medicare payment is based on the discipline and location of the clinician, who must be operating within the scope of practice under state law to receive reimbursement for telemedicine services (Wholey et al., 2003). A more comprehensive approach to Medicare and Medicaid coverage and payment policy is needed to support technology implementation.

Numerous options have been proposed for facilitating the use of telemedicine while maintaining appropriate regulatory protections. These include issuance of a national telemedicine license, with telehealth being viewed as interstate commerce (Bashshur et al., 1994; IOM, 1996; NRC, 2000; Sanders et al., 1995) and the development and widespread adoption of model state laws and regulations pertaining to telemedicine. Evaluation of these options is beyond the scope of this report, but this issue should be addressed by the National Coordinator for Health Information Technology.

> ***Key Finding 4.*** *Telehealth warrants special attention to facilitate use while maintaining appropriate regulatory protections. Some changes in government regulatory processes and health insurance programs may be desirable, but a detailed analysis of current practices for purposes of identifying barriers to telehealth has yet to be conducted. The Office of the National Coordinator for Health Information Technology might provide leadership and coordination for such work.*

Financial Assistance for EHRs

If rural communities are to benefit from the NHII, financial assistance from the federal government will be required. Most rural health care is provided in small ambulatory practice settings and small hospitals, many of which are financially fragile and have limited access to capital for investing in EHRs (see Chapter 5). Rural health systems are also more dependent than urban systems on public payment programs, such as Medicaid, safety net grant programs for community and rural health clinics, and Medicare. In rural areas, such as Indian reservations, the federal government may also be the dominant provider of services.

The federal government should pursue multiple strategies to assist rural providers in implementing EHRs. One size will not fit all. The committee recommends a four-pronged approach.

First, the federal government should accelerate the adoption of EHRs by federally owned health care organizations serving rural areas, such as the Indian Health Service. Building on the excellent accomplishments of the Veterans Health Administration (VHA), which has already adopted EHRs (Duncan et al., 1995), emphasis should be placed on rapid deployment of this technology to Indian Health Service providers (e.g., hospitals, clinics, nursing homes). Greater efforts should also be undertaken to make the VHA's software (i.e., VISTA) available to and usable by private-sector providers (e.g., small hospitals) in rural areas.

Second, HRSA, which administers the community health center and rural health clinic programs, should provide resources and technical assistance to these ambulatory providers for the acquisition and use of EHRs. HRSA should work collaboratively with private-sector organizations, such as the American Academy of Family Physicians (AAFP), which is sponsoring an initiative to assist small and medium-sized offices of family practitioners with the purchase and implementation of EHRs and the training and technical assistance required to incorporate the technology into their practice (AAFP, 2003). AAFP's initiative includes both the Open EHR Pilot Project, a small-scale phase 1 project to study and promote the transition to a paperless office and the use of EHRs, and the Doctors Office Quality Information Technology project, designed to assist physicians' offices in migrating from paper to EHRs, storing health information electronically, and using computer-generated decision support tools (AAFP, 2003).

Third, consistent with the recommendations of other IOM committees (IOM, 2002a), this committee encourages the Centers for Medicare and Medicaid Services (CMS), which administers the Medicare program, to consider providing modest financial incentives to providers for investing in EHRs. Other public and private purchasers should do the same. Financial incentives to providers should be conditional upon the acquisition and use of EHRs that possess key capabilities necessary for the provision of high-quality care (IOM, 2003c,d). The bulk of costs and behavior changes is the responsibility of providers, while the bulk of benefits accrues to patients and insurers. As a major insurer, the federal government has every reason to speed the transition to EHRs.

Fourth, all public and private purchasers should reexamine their benefit and payment policies to ensure adequate coverage and payment for telemedicine and other services delivered electronically. Adequate payment for these services will result in a more favorable return on investment in ICT. Lack of reimbursement for telemedicine services has likely been the chief economic issue hindering their broad acceptance and utilization (Wholey et al., 2003).

> **Recommendation 10. Congress should provide appropriate direction and financial resources to assist rural providers in converting to electronic health records over the next 5 years. Working collaboratively with the Office of the National Coordinator for Health Information Technology:**
>
> • **The Indian Health Service should develop a strategy for transitioning all of its provider sites (including those operated by tribal governments under the Self-Determination Act) from paper to electronic health records.**
> • **The Health Resources and Services Administration should develop a strategy for transitioning community health centers, rural health clinics, critical access hospitals, and other rural providers from paper to electronic health records.**
> • **The Centers for Medicare and Medicaid Services and the state governments should consider providing financial rewards to providers participating in Medicare or Medicaid programs that invest in electronic health records. These two large public insurance programs should work together to reexamine their benefit and payment programs to ensure appropriate coverage of telehealth and other health services delivered electronically.**

ICT Collaborations and Demonstrations in Rural Areas

The ultimate goal is to establish a national and even global health information infrastructure that allows for the exchange of patient data between authorized users (e.g., personal physicians) in a secure environment. However, the NHII will likely be built community by community, with local or regional health information infrastructures adhering to national data standards. Rural communities should be actively engaged in this developmental work to establish local networks for the exchange of data. Moreover, local NHII efforts need to be cross-linked to the information infrastructure projects of other sectors (e.g., education, agriculture) to build on existing resources and integrate new technology.

There are notable examples of community- or statewide efforts to establish data exchange networks. For example, in the private sector, the Indiana Network for Patient Care, developed with leadership from the Regenstrief Institute, is a network of 13 acute care hospitals in Indianapolis and 20 percent of outpatient physician practices (Overhage, 2003). Participating organizations pay a monthly fee for access to selected electronic information that forms the basis for an "operational communitywide electronic medical record," including reports from emergency room visits, laboratory results, admission notes/discharge summaries, operative reports, radiology reports, surgical pathology reports, inpatient medications, immunizations, and a tumor registry (Overhage, 2003). Each health care provider retains its patients' information in its organization's database; however, selected information in those datasets can be shared among organizations through use of a Global Patient Index (Overhage, 2003). The Indiana Network for Patient Care not only allows for the secure storage and exchange of clinical information, but also provides clinical decision support and population health surveillance and reporting. Other examples of data exchange networks include the CareScience system in Santa Barbara, California (Carescience, 2003), Winona Health Online in Minnesota (Chin, 2002), and the New England Health Exchange Network in Waltham, Massachusetts (Glaser et al., 2003). Others are at various stages of development.

Establishing community- or statewide information infrastructures requires a high degree of collaboration across the public and private sectors. There are steps that can be taken now to foster such collaboration. First, Congress should remove regulatory barriers that may impede collaboration around ICT issues in rural communities. Concern has been raised that provisions under the Social Security Act, Section 1877, and subsequent amendments (i.e., "Stark I" and "Stark II"), originally intended to restrict physicians from making referrals to laboratories in which the referring physician has an ownership or other financial stake, may have the unintended consequence of impeding collaborative arrangements between providers (e.g., hospitals and physicians) to establish EHRs (Personal communication, G. Greenberg, May 6, 2004; Jacobs, 2004). Further clarification of the intent of the law and possibly the creation of a safe harbor for ICT-related collaboration would be advisable.

In addition, the federal government should provide financial support to a limited number of rural communities for the establishment of communitywide health information infrastructures. Efforts to this end are already under way. AHRQ will be providing $139 million in grants to fund health information technology (HIT) development projects in three categories. The first is promoting access to HIT through grants to communities, hospitals, providers, and health care systems. These grants are spread across 38 states, with a special focus on small and rural hospitals and communities.

Second is developing statewide and regional networks through 5-year contracts, recently awarded to Colorado, Indiana, Rhode Island, Tennessee, and Utah. Third is establishing a National HIT Resource Center that will provide technical assistance, maintain a repository of best practices, and disseminate useful tools to help with technology adoption. The grant to develop the center was awarded to the University of Chicago (AHRQ, 2004b). Award of the HIT grants (community and statewide) requires the awardees to develop a comprehensive plan encompassing technology adoption, partnerships for interconnections, methods for overcoming barriers to adoption, staff responsibilities, technical assistance needed, an implementation timeline, budget, and measures for ongoing project evaluation (AHRQ, 2003b). The data exchange networks in rural areas are to include academic health centers and providers in urban areas.

The committee applauds these efforts, but is concerned that current funding may be inadequate to fully develop the NHII. Additional funding to rural and frontier areas will be needed to build infrastructure on a national scale. The committee encourages Congress to provide adequate resources to continue the award of grants at both the community and state levels to complete the development of the NHII. The HIT projects noted above and all new projects should incorporate a follow-on phase upon project completion that focuses on interconnections to the larger structure of the NHII. For regions with large rural areas, especially those with large frontier areas, follow-on plans may be coordinated at the state level.

> **Recommendation 11. The Agency for Healthcare Research and Quality's Health Information Technology Program should be expanded. Adequate resources should be provided to allow the agency to sponsor developmental programs for information and communications technology in five rural areas. Communities should be selected from across the range of rural environments, including frontier areas. The 5-year developmental programs should commence in fiscal year 2006 and result in the establishment of state-of-the-art information and communications technology infrastructure that is accessible to all providers and all consumers in those communities.**

It should also be noted that building an ICT infrastructure must be an integral component of the health system reform demonstrations recommended in Chapter 2. As discussed in Chapter 1, the committee endorses the "bottom-up" approach to health system reform proposed in the earlier IOM report *Fostering Rapid Advances in Health Care: Learning from System*

Demonstrations (IOM, 2003a). Chapter 2 recommended a set of demonstration projects in those communities to test alternative approaches to restructuring the health systems in rural communities to address both population and personal health care needs in a more integrated fashion, and to redesign finance and delivery system to achieve those objectives. Adequate ICT capabilities and supports will be critical to these demonstrations as well.

Ongoing Educational Assistance

Rural communities, like urban areas, are embarking on a period of enormous change. Communities will need both technical and educational assistance to make this transition smoothly and successfully. The technical challenges are sizable, but so, too, are the human and organizational issues involved.

A growing body of literature documents that human and organizational factors play a significant role in the delays being seen in the widespread adoption of ICT (Clayton et al., 2003; Perednia and Allen, 1995). Factors contributing to resistance to ICT adoption include computer anxiety (Gamm et al., 1998), increased time to enter orders and patient histories compared with paper-based methods (Krall, 1995; Sittig et al., 1999), decreased patient–physician interaction (Gadd and Penrod, 2000; Gamm et al., 1998), inability to integrate applications into the physician's workflow (Sittig et al., 1999), and decreased educational opportunities (Ash et al., 1999). The National Advisory Committee on Rural Health and Human Services (NACRHHS, 2003) has noted that health care professional training programs have failed to incorporate technology skill development into their curricula in any meaningful way. Clinicians are forced to learn and adapt on the job, which greatly slows the diffusion of technologies for improving care. Health professionals need ongoing, lifelong technology training and skill development, with particular emphasis on telehealth technologies (Nesbitt et al., 2004).

Overcoming personal and cultural challenges to technology diffusion is possible through education and communication addressing the major influences on adoption: the relative advantages of newer over existing technologies; the degree to which technologies are perceived to be compatible with the values, experiences, and needs of their users; concerns related to the complexity of understanding and using the technologies; the degree to which providers can experiment with the technologies on a limited basis; and the observability of the results of an innovation. Each rural community will need a plan for phasing in ICT applications, starting with a few of the most basic applications (e.g., drug interaction checking, order entry, laboratory and radiology test results), followed by applications that require more fundamental changes in care processes and relationships among clinicians and between clinicians and patients (e.g., telemedicine consultation).

Because the delivery of health care services involves many disciplines (e.g., clinicians, ancillary support personnel, technical specialists, and administrative personnel) and organizations (e.g., primary care offices, clinics, hospitals, nursing homes, tertiary care hospitals, and specialty services outside the community), it will be important to pursue a coordinated approach to technology adoption that builds on existing networks. This point is particularly applicable to rural communities. Networking[8] among rural providers and with urban organizations has been central to building more stable rural health care delivery systems and addressing some of the workforce supply issues faced by rural areas. By coalescing voluntarily into cooperatives, alliances, consortia, or networks, rural providers can often reduce their costs; manage their scarce resources; and increase their bargaining position, including that related to the purchase, training, and implementation of health ICT systems (Goldsmith et al., 1997). The provider relationships developed through networks mirror the relationships needed for the electronic information sharing and data exchange associated with EHRs and telemedicine technologies. Roughly one-third to one-half of rural providers are already involved in an alliance of some sort (Moscovice et al., 2003). Continued development of these networks would more fully support the rural health care delivery system, the adoption of ICT among local providers, and interconnections with the NHII.

Strong clinical and administrative leadership will also be important to the implementation of ICT. Achieving an effective level of teamwork for technology implementation requires regular interaction, cooperation, and collaboration among the different providers involved. If urban organizations are part of the network, their senior management and clinicians must

---

[8] The term "rural health network" refers to a formal organizational arrangement among rural health care providers (and possibly insurers and social service providers) that uses the resources of more than one existing organization and specifies the objectives and methods by which various collaborative functions will be achieved (Moscovice et al., 1997). Networks can be vertical or horizontal or both. In such networks, the organizational arrangement is formal (i.e., explicit and legal), membership is specified, resources are committed by members (e.g., time, money), and the network is purposeful (e.g., sharing or integrating services).

be educated about the realities of the rural health care environment and the needs of rural clinicians in moving forward with ICT. Both rural and urban provider facilities must have input into the strategic processes and development of a comprehensive, viable plan for implementing EHRs and telemedicine technologies progressively over time.

Another important aspect of the adoption of ICT is obtaining the commitment of clinicians to use the technologies and to provide ongoing feedback regarding any hesitations or problems associated with their use. Important as well is the identification of a technology champion to lead and support the implementation and use of ICT at the provider level. Individual practice providers and those belonging to networks in rural areas also should participate in quality improvement initiatives linking them to regional organizations that can further support them in their efforts to incorporate ICT.

The National Library of Medicine and the National Network of Libraries of Medicine have an extensive track record of providing educational resources to communities (NLM, 2004b). Among the lessons learned from their outreach projects for health professionals is that the barriers to the adoption of ICT are multidimensional, but that the process of changing health professionals' information habits is facilitated by repeated contact, including hands-on training, and by awareness that there is a human resource that can be consulted as questions and problems arise (Wallingford et al., 1996).

Recommendation 12. The National Library of Medicine, in collaboration with the Office of the National Coordinator for Health Information Technology and the Agency for Healthcare Research and Quality, should establish regional information and communications technology/telehealth resource centers that are interconnected with the National Network of Libraries of Medicine. These resource centers should provide a full spectrum of services, including the following:

  • **Information resources for health professionals and consumers, including access to online information sources and technical assistance with online applications, such as distance monitoring.**
  • **Lifelong educational programs for health care professionals.**
  • **An on-call resource center to assist communities in resolving technical, organizational, clinical, financial, and legal questions related to information and communications technology.**

REFERENCES

AAFP (American Academy of Family Physicians). 2003. *Current Projects*. [Online]. Available: http://www.aafp.org/x24654.xml [accessed June 14, 2004].

ACP (American College of Physicians). 2003. *Information Rx Project*. [Online]. Available: http://foundation.acponline.org/healthcom/info_rx.htm [accessed June 29, 2004].

AHRQ (Agency for Healthcare Research and Quality). 2003a. *U.S. Department of Health and Human Services FY 2004 Budget in Brief*. [Online]. Available: http://www.hhs.gov/budget/04budget/fy2004bib.pdf [accessed June 28, 2004].

AHRQ. 2003b. *Transforming Healthcare Quality through Information Technology—Planning Grants*. [Online]. Available: http://grants.nih.gov/grants/guide/rfa-files/RFA-HS-04-010.html [accessed April 27, 2004].

AHRQ. 2004a. *Testimony on the President's Fiscal Year 2004 Budget Request for AHRQ*. [Online]. Available: http://www.ahrq.gov/about/cj2004/cjtest05.htm [accessed June 29, 2004].

AHRQ. 2004b. *HHS Awards $139 Million to Drive Adoption of Health Information Technology*. [Online]. Available: http://www.ahrq.gov/news/press/pr2004/hhshitpr.htm [accessed October 19, 2004].

Allen D, Bowersox J, Jones GG. 1997. Telesurgery, telepresence, telementoring, telerobotics. *Telemedicine Today* 5(3):18–20, 25.

Allen KC. 2001. *Advanced Telecommunications in Rural America*. [Online]. Available: http://www.its.bldrdoc.gov/tpr/2000/its_t/adv_tele/adv_tele.html [accessed July 7, 2004].

Anderson JG. 2001a. Cyberhealthcare: Reshaping the physician-patient relationship. *M.D. Computing: Computers in Medical Practice* 18(1):21–22.

Anderson JG. 2001b. *How the Internet is Transforming the Physician-Patient Relationship*. [Online]. Available: http://www.medscape.com/viewarticle/415047_print [accessed July 7, 2004].

Anderson JG, Horvath J. 2002. *Chronic Conditions: Making the Case for Ongoing Care*. Baltimore, MD: Johns Hopkins University and The Robert Wood Johnson Foundation.

Appel PR, Bleiberg J, Noiseux J. 2002. Self-regulation training for chronic pain: Can it be done effectively by telemedicine? *Telemedicine Journal and e-Health* 8(4):361–368.

Armstrong ML, Frueh S. 2002. *Telecommunications for Nurses: Providing Successful Distance Education and Telehealth*. New York: Springer Publishing Co.

Ash JS, Gorman PN, Hersh WR, Poulsen SB, Lavelle M. 1999. *Perceptions of House Officers Who Use Physician Order Entry*. Paper presented at the meeting of the Proceedings of Annual American Medical Informatics Association Symposium. Bethesda, MD: American Medical Informatics Association.

Baigent MF, Lloyd CJ, Kavanagh SJ, Ben-Tovim DI, Yellowlees PM, Kalucy RS, Bond MJ. 1997. Telepsychiatry: "Tele" yes, but what about the "psychiatry"? *Journal of Telemedicine and Telecare* 3(Supplement 1):3–5.

Balas EA, Boren SA, Hicks LL, Chinko AM, Stephenson K. 1998. Effect of linking practice data to published evidence: A randomized controlled trial of clinical direct reports. *Medical Care* 36(1):79–87.

Bashshur RL, Homan RK, Smith DG. 1994. Beyond the uninsured: Problems in access to care. *Medical Care* 32(5):409–419.

BCG (The Boston Consulting Group). 2003. *E-Health's Influence Continues to Grow as Use of the Internet by Physicians and Patients Increases.* [Online]. Available: http://www.bcg.com/publications/publication_view.jsp?pubID=913&language=English [accessed July 31, 2004].

Becher EC, Chassin MR. 2001. Improving quality, minimizing error: Making it happen. *Health Affairs* 20(5):164–179.

Bennett J. 2002 (December 26). Patients skip the waiting room for virtual visits to the doctor. *Wall Street Journal.* P. A4.

Berendt M, Schaefer B, Heglund MJ, Bardin C. 2001. Telehealth for effective disease state management. *Home Care Provider* 6(2):67–72.

Bodenheimer T, Wagner EH, Grumbach K. 2002. Improving primary care for patients with chronic illness: The chronic care model Part 2. *Journal of the American Medical Association* 288(15):1909–1914.

Brailer DJ. 2003. *Use and Adoption of Computer-based Patient Records in the United States: A Review and Update.* Commissioned paper for the IOM Committee on Data Standards for Patient Safety. Washington, DC.

Breslow MJ. 2000. ICU telemedicine: Organization and communication. *Critical Care Clinics* 16(4):707–722.

Burke M, Evans WD. 2003. *Information Technology Survey Report for the Turning Point National Excellence Collaborative for Information Technology.* [Online]. Available: http://www.turningpointprogram.org/Pages/IT%20Survey%20Report.pdf [accessed June 14, 2004].

Carescience. 2003. *Santa Barbara County Care Data Exchange.* [Online]. Available: http://www.carescience.com/healthcare_providers/cde/care_data_exchange_santabarbara_cde.shtml [accessed July 7, 2004].

Casal CR, Schoute F, Prasad R. 2004. *Evolution Towards Fourth Generation Mobile Multimedia Communication.* [Online]. Available: http://www.ubicom.tudelft.nl/MMC/Docs/paper38.pdf [accessed July 7, 2004].

Castelnuovo G, Gaggioli A, Riva G. 2001. *The Emergence of e-Therapy in Mental Health Care.* Amsterdam, NE, Washington, DC: IOS Press. Pp. 229, 252.

Celi LA, Hassan E, Marquardt C. 2001. The EICU: It's not just telemedicine. *Critical Care Medicine* 29(8 Supplement):N183–N189.

Chetney R. 2002. Interactive home telehealth: Moving from cost savings to reimbursement. Creative, proactive strategies help agencies turn telehealth into a revenue generator. *Telemedicine Today* 9(3):19–20.

Chin T. 2002. *The Winona Project: Developing an Electronic Link.* [Online]. Available: http://www.ama-assn.org/amednews/2002/03/11/bisa0311.htm [accessed July 7, 2004].

CIT (Center for Information Therapy). 2004. *Center for Information Therapy* (homepage). [Online]. Available: http://www.informationtherapy.org/cit.html [accessed June 29, 2004].

Clayton PD, Narus SP, Huff SM, Pryor TA, Haug PJ, Larkin T, Matney S, Evans RS, Rocha BH, Bowes WA, Holston FT, Gundersen ML. 2003. Building a comprehensive clinical information system from components: The approach at InterMountain. *Methods of Information in Medicine* 41:1–7.

Covell D, Uman G, Manning P. 1985. Information needs in office practice: Are they being met? *Annals of Internal Medicine* 103(4):596–599.

Cummings DM, Morrissey S, Barondes MJ. 2001. Screening for diabetic retinopathy in rural areas: The potential of telemedicine. *Journal of Rural Health* 17(1):25–31.

D'Alessandro DM, D'Alessandro MP, Galvin JR, Kash JB, Wakefield DS, Erkonen WE. 1988. Barriers to rural physician use of a digital health sciences library. *Bulletin of the Medical Library Association* 86(4):583–593.

Davidson P. 2004 (July 15). Inventive wireless providers go rural. *USA Today.* P. Money1B.

Duesing A. 2002. Community connections in off-campus outreach services. *Journal of Library Administration* 37(1/2):269–278.

Duncan RP, Seccombe K, Amey C. 1995. Changes in health insurance coverage within rural and urban environments—1977 to 1987. *Journal of Rural Health* 11(3):169–176.

Eadie LH, Seifalian AM, Davidson BR. 2003. Telemedicine in surgery. *British Journal of Surgery* 90(6):647–658.

Field MJ, Grigsby J. 2002. Telemedicine and remote patient monitoring. *Journal of the American Medical Association* 288(4):423–425.

Fox S, Fallows D. 2003. *Internet Health Resources.* Washington, DC: Pew Internet and American Life Project.

Gadd CS, Penrod LE. 2000. *Dichotomy Between Physicians' and Patients' Attitudes Regarding EMR Use During Outpatient Encounters.* Paper presented at the meeting of the Proceeding of American Medical Informatics Symposium. Bethesda, MD: American Medical Informatics Association.

Gamm LD, Barsukiewicz CK, Dansky KH, Vasey JJ, Bisordi JE, Thompson PC. 1998. Pre- and post-control model research on end-users' satisfaction with an electronic medical record: Preliminary results. *Proceeding of American Medical Informatics Symposium* 225–229.

Glaser JP, DeBor G, Schultz L. 2003. New England healthcare EDI network. *Journal of Health Information Management* 17(4).

Glick TH, Moore GT. 2001. Time to learn: The outlook for renewal of patient-centered education in the digital age. *Medical Education* 35(5):505–509.

Goldsmith HF, Wagenfeld MO, Manderscheid RW, Stiles D. 1997. Specialty mental health services in metropolitan and nonmetropolitan areas: 1983 and 1990. *Administration and Policy in Mental Health* 24(6):475–488.

Griffiths KM, Christensen H. 2000. Quality of web-based information on treatment of depression: Cross sectional survey. *British Medical Journal* 321(7275):1511–1515.

Guard R, Fredericka TM, Kroll S, Marine S, Roddy C, Steiner T, Wentz S. 2000. Health care, information needs, and outreach: Reaching Ohio's rural citizens. *Bulletin of the Medical Library Association* 88(4):374–381.

Haas SW. 2001. *An Overview of State and Federal Universal Service/Access Support Mechanisms and Administration in the United States.* [Online]. Available: http://www.wallman.com/pdfs_etc/ptc_2002.doc [accessed September 15, 2004].

Hart LG, Salsberg E, Phillips DM, Lishner DM. 2002. Rural health care providers in the United States. *Journal of Rural Health* 18(Supplement):211–232.

Hartley D, Ziller E, MacDonald C. 2002. *Diabetes and the Rural Safety Net:* Portland, ME: Maine Rural Health Research Center, University of Southern Maine.

Hashimoto S, Shirato H, Kaneko K, Ooshio W, Nishioka T, Miyasaka K. 2001. Clinical efficacy of telemedicine in emergency radiotherapy for malignant spinal cord compression. *Journal of Digital Imaging* 14(3):124–130.

Haskins PA, Ellis DG, Mayrose J. 2002. Predicted utilization of emergency medical services telemedicine in decreasing ambulance transports. *Prehospital Emergency Care* 6(4):445–448.

Hassol A, Gaumer G, Irvin C, Grigsby J, Mintzer C, Puskin D. 1997a. Rural telemedicine data/image transfer methods and purposes of interactive video sessions. *Journal of the American Medical Informatics Association* 4(1):36–37.

Hassol A, Irvin C, Gaumer G, Puskin D, Mintzer C, Grigsby J. 1997b. Rural applications of telemedicine. *Telemedicine Journal and e-Health* 3(3):215–225.

Helms, WD. 2001. *Issues and Research*. [Online]. Available: http://www.ahcpr.gov/news/ulp/rural/ulprurl9.htm [accessed June 28, 2004].

Hilty DM, Liu W, Marks SL, Callahan EJ. 2003. Effectiveness of telepsychiatry: A review. *Canadian Psychiatric Association (Bulletin)*. [Online]. Available: http://www.cpa-apc.org/publications/archives/bulletin/2003/october/hilty.asp [accessed March 2004].

Homan JM. 2002. *The Role of Librarians in Reducing Medical Errors*. [Online]. Available: http://www.healthleaders.com/news/feature1.php?contentid=38058 [accessed January 29, 2004].

IHS (Indian Health Service). 2000. *Indian Health Service Fiscal Year 2001 Budget 9.25% Increase Proposed*. [Online]. Available: http://www.ihs.gov/PublicInfo/PublicAffairs/PressReleases/PressRelease2000/BudgetFY2001.asp [accessed June 29, 2004].

IOM (Institute of Medicine). 1996. *Telemedicine: A Guide to Assessing Telecommunications in Health Care*. Washington, DC: National Academy Press.

IOM. 1997. *The Computer-Based Patient Record*. Washington, DC: National Academy Press.

IOM. 2001a. *Crossing the Quality Chasm: A New Health System for the 21st Century*. Washington, DC: National Academy Press.

IOM. 2001b. *Improving the Quality of Long Term Care*. Washington, DC: National Academy Press.

IOM. 2002a. *Leadership by Example: Coordinating Government Roles in Improving Health Care Quality*. Washington, DC: The National Academies Press.

IOM. 2002b. *Unequal Treatment: Confronting Racial and Ethnic Disparities in Health Care*. Washington, DC: The National Academies Press.

IOM. 2003a. *Fostering Rapid Advances in Health Care: Learning from System Demononstrations*. Washington, DC: The National Academies Press.

IOM. 2003b. *The Future of the Public's Health in the 21st Century*. Washington, DC: The National Academies Press.

IOM. 2003c. *Letter Report: Key Capabilities of an Electronic Health Record System*. Washington, DC: The National Academies Press.

IOM. 2003d. *Patient Safety: Achieving a New Standard for Care*. Washington, DC: The National Academies Press.

IOM. 2003e. *Priority Areas for National Action: Transforming Health Care Quality*. Washington, DC: The National Academies Press.

IOM. 2004. *Health Literacy: A Prescription to End Confusion*. Washington, DC: The National Academies Press.

Jacobs RO. 2004. *Stark Handbook (Phase I and II)*. St Petersburg, FL: Holland and Knight.

James B. 2003. Information system concepts for quality measurement. *Medical Care* 41(Supplement 1)I-71–I-79.

Javitt JC. 2004 (May 25). Perspective: How to succeed in health information technology. *Health Affairs*. Web exclusive. [Online]. Available: http://content.healthaffairs.org/cgi/reprint/hlthaff.w4.321v1?maxtoshow=&HITS=10&hits=10&RESULTFORMAT=&fulltext=%22national+health+information+infrastructure%22&andorexactfulltext=and&searchid=1088446717542_1681&stored_search=&FIRSTINDEX= 0&resourcetype= 1&journalcode=healthaff [accessed June 2004].

Jenkins RL, White P. 2001. Telehealth Advancing Nursing Practice. *Nursing Outlook* 49(2):100–105.

Jennett PA, Affleck Hall L, Hailey D, Ohinmaa A, Anderson C, Thomas R, Young B, Lorenzetti D, Scott RE. 2003. The socio-economic impact of telehealth: A systematic review. *Journal of Telemedicine and Telecare* 9(6):311–320.

Jerome RN, Giuse NB, Gish KW, Sathe NA, Dietrich MS. 2001. Information needs of clinical teams: Analysis of questions received by the clinical information consult service. *Bulletin of the Medical Library Association* 89(2):177–185.

Johnson KB, Ravert RD, Everton A. 2001. Hopkins teen central: Assessment of an Internet-based support system for children with cystic fibrosis. *Pediatrics* 107(2):E24.

Johnston B, Wheeler L, Deuser J, Sousa KH. 2000. Outcomes of the Kaiser Permanente tele-home health research project. *Archives of Family Medicine* 9(1):40–45.

Keeling P, Hughes D, Price L, Shaw S, Barton A. 2003. Safety and feasibility of prehospital thrombolysis carried out by paramedics. *British Medical Journal* 327(7405):27–28.

Kennedy C, Yellowlees P. 2000. A community-based approach to the evaluation of health outcomes and costs for telepsychiatry in a rural population: Preliminary results. *Journal of Telemedicine and Telecare* 6(Supplement 1):S155–157.

Kibee D. 2004. *Health Information Technology Adoption in Rural Family Practice*. Presentation at the Workshop on the Future of Rural Health: A Quality Focus (March 1–2, 2004). Washington, DC.

Kim MI, Johnson KB. 2002. Personal health records: Evaluation of functionality and utility. *Journal of the American Medical Informatics Association* 9(2):171–180.

King DN. 1987. Contribution of hospital library services: A study. *Bulletin of the Medical Library Association* 75(4):269–299.

Klein MS, Ross FV, Adams DL, Gilbert CM. 1994. Effect of online literature searching on length of stay and patient care costs. *Academic Medicine* 69(6):489–495.

Kobb R, Hoffman N, Lodge R, Kline S. 2003. Enhancing elder chronic care through technology and care coordination: Report from a pilot. *Telemedicine Journal and e-Health* 9(2):189–195.

Kobza L, Scheurich A. 2000. The impact of telemedicine on outcomes of chronic wounds in the home care setting. *Ostomy/Wound Management* 46(10):48–53.

Krall MA. 1995. *Acceptance and Performance by Clinicians Using an Ambulatory Electronic Medical Record in an HMO.* Paper presented at the Proceedings of the Nineteenth Symposium of Computer Applications in Medical Care. Bethesda, MD: American Medical Informatics Association.

LaMonte MP, Bahouth MN, Hu P, Pathan MY, Yarbrough KL, Gunawardane R, Crarey P, Page W. 2003. Telemedicine for acute stroke: Triumphs and pitfalls. *Stroke* 34(3):725–728.

Lee JK, Renner JB, Saunders BF, Stamford PP, Bickford TR, Johnston RE, Hsaio HS, Phillips ML. 1998. Effect of real-time teleradiology on the practice of the emergency department physician in a rural setting: Initial experience. *Academic Radiology* 5(8):533–538.

Levine SR, Gorman M. 1999. Telestroke: The application of telemedicine for stroke. *Stroke* 30(2):464–469.

Liederman EM, Morefield CS. 2003. Web messaging: A new tool for patient-physician communication. *Journal of the American Medical Informatics Association* 10(3):260–270.

Liesenfeld B, Kohner E, Piehmeier W, Kluthe W, Aldington S, Porta M, Bek T, Obermaier M, Mayer H, Mann G, Holle R, Hepp KD. 2000. A telemedical approach to the screening of diabetic retinopathy: Digital fundus photography. *Diabetes Care* 23(3):345–348.

Lindberg DA, Siegel ER, Rapp BA, Wallingford KT, Wilson SR. 1993. Use of MEDLINE by physicians for clinical problem solving. *Journal of the American Medical Association* 269(24):3124–3129.

Lorence DP, Spink A, Richards MA. 2002. EPR adoption and dual record maintenance in the U.S.: Assessing variation in medical systems infrastructure. *Journal of Medical Systems* 26(5):357–367.

Lumpkin, JR. 2000. *Report on the Uniform Data Standards for Patient Medical Record Information.* [Online]. Available: http://www.ncvhs.hhs.gov/hipaa000706.pdf [accessed July 7, 2004].

Madden M, Raine L. 2003. *America's Online Pursuits: The Changing Picture of Who's Online and What They Do.* Washington, DC: Pew Internet and American Life Project.

Marcin JP, Nesbitt TS, Kallas HJ, Struve SN, Traugott CA, Dimand RJ. 2004. Use of telemedicine to provide pediatric critical care inpatient consultations to underserved rural Northern California. *Journal of Pediatrics* 144(3):375–380.

Markle Foundation. 2003. *The Steering Group: Key Themes and Guiding Principles.* [Online]. Available: http://www.markle.org/downloadable_assets/sg_final.pdf [accessed July 7, 2004].

Marshall JG. 1992. The impact of the hospital library on clincial decision making: The Rochester Study. *Bulletin of the Medical Library Association* 80(2):169–178.

Matherlee K. 2001. *Mission Possible?: Maintaining the Safety Net in Urban and Rural Colorado.* Washington, DC: National Health Policy Forum.

Mayo Clinic. 2004. *MayoClinic.com.* [Online]. Available: http://www.mayoclinic.com/ [accessed May 14, 2004].

McCloskey KM. 2000. Library outreach: Addressing Utah's "digital divide." *Bulletin of the Medical Library Association* 88(4):367–373.

McGowan JJ. 2000. Health information outreach: The land-grant mission. *Bulletin of the Medical Library Association* 88(4):355–361.

McLaren P, Yellowlees PM, Wootton R. 2003. *Conclusion.* Wootton R, Yellowlees PM, McLaren P, eds. London, UK: Royal Society of Medicine Press. Pp. 349–354.

McMahon K, Salant P. 1999. Strategic planning for telecommunications in rural communities. *Rural Development Perspectives* 14(3):2–7.

Melzner SM, Grossman DC, Hart LG, Rosenblatt RA. 1997. Hospital services for rural children in Washington state. *Pediatrics* 99(2):196–203.

Moscovice I, Casey, M, and Krein, S. 1997. *Rural Managed Care: Patterns and Prospects.* Minneapolis, MN: Rural Health Research Center, University of Minnesota.

Moscovice I, Gregg W, Lewerenz E. 2003 (June). *Rural Health Networks: Evolving Organizational Forms and Functions.* Minneapolis, MN: Rural Health Research Center.

Mueller KJ, Coburn A, Cordes S, Crittenden R, Hart JP, McBride T, Myers W. 1999. The changing landscape of health care financing and delivery: How are rural communities and providers responding? *The Milbank Quarterly* 77(4):485–509.

Mueller KJ, Stoner JA, Shambaugh-Miller MD, Lucas WO, Pol LG. 2003. Method for identifying places in rural America at risk of not being able to support adequate health services. *Journal of Rural Health* 19(4):450–460.

NACRHHS (National Advisory Committee on Rural Health and Human Services). 2000. *Rural Public Health: Issues and Considerations.* Washington, DC: U.S. Department of Health and Human Services.

NACRHHS. 2003. *Health Care Quality: The Rural Context.* Washington, DC: U.S. Department of Health and Human Services.

NCHC (National Coalition on Health Care). 2002. *Accelerating Change Today.* Washington, DC: National Coalition on Health Care.

NCSL (National Conference of State Legislatures). 2000 (August). *Emergency Medical Services in Rural Areas: How Can States Ensure Their Effectiveness?* [Online]. Available: http://www.ncsl.org/programs/health/Forum/ruralems.htm [accessed May 2004].

NCVHS (National Committee on Vital and Health Statistics). 2001. *Information for Health: A Strategy for Building the National Health Information Infrastructure.* Washington, DC: U.S. Department of Health and Human Services.

Nelson EL, Barnard M, Cain S. 2003. Treating childhood depression over videoconferencing. *Telemedicine Journal and e-Health* 9(1):49–55.

Nesbitt TS, Marcin JP. 2002. Clinical outcomes: The impact of telemedicine. *Telemedicine Journal and e-Health* 8(2):214.

Nesbitt TS, Jerant A, Balsbaugh T. 2002. Equipping primary care physicians for the digital age: The Internet, online education, handheld computers, and telemedicine. *The Western Journal of Medicine* 176(2):116–120.

Nesbitt TS, Tran TP, Katz J. 2004. *Continuing Education for Telemedicine Programs: The UC Davis Health System Teaching Model.* Whitten P, Cook D, eds. San Francisco, CA: Jossey-Bass.

NLM (National Library of Medicine). 2004a. *Medline Plus.* [Online]. Available: http://medlineplus.gov/ [accessed May 14, 2004].

NLM. 2004b. *Fact Sheet: National Network of Libraries of Medicine.* [Online]. Available: http://www.nlm.nih.gov/pubs/factsheets/nnlm.html [accessed June 29, 2004].

NRC (National Research Council). 2000. *Networking Health.* Washington, DC: National Academy Press.

OMB (Office of Management and Budget). 2000. *Standards for Defining Metropolitan and Micropolitan Statistical Areas.* [Online]. Available: http://www.census.gov/ population/www/estimates/00-32997.pdf.

ORHP (Office of Rural Health Policy). 2002. *One Department Serving Rural America.* Washington, DC: U.S. Department of Health and Human Services.

OTP (Office of Technology Policy). 2004. *Innovation, Demand, and Investment in Telehealth.* Washington, DC: U.S. Department of Commerce.

Overhage M. 2003. *Enhancing Public Health, Healthcare System, and Clinician Preparedness: Strategies to Promote Coordination and Communication.* Washington, DC: The Indiana Network for Patient Care.

Patricoski C, Ferguson AS. 2003. ECG acquisition using telemedicine in Alaska. *Alaska Medicine* 45(3):60–63.

Patterson V, Hoque F, Vassallo D. 2001. Store-and-forward teleneurology in developing countries. *Journal of Telemedicine and Telecare* 7(Supplement 1):52–53.

Perednia DA, Allen A. 1995. Telemedicine technology and clinical applications. *The Journal of the American Medical Association* 273(6):483–488.

PHPPO (Public Health Practice Program Office). 2002. *Health Alert Network.* [Online]. Available: http://www.phppo.cdc.gov/HAN/Index.asp [accessed June 27, 2004].

Pifalo V. 2000. The evolution of rural outreach from package library to grateful med: Introduction to the symposium. *Bulletin of the Medical Library Association* 88(4):339–345.

Quintero RA, Munoz H, Pommer R, Diaz C, Bornick PW, Allen MH. 2002. Operative fetoscopy via telesurgery. *Ultrasound in Obstetrics and Gynecology* 20(4):390–391.

Raikin SM, Bley LA, Leb RB. 1999. Emerging technology: Remote analysis of traumatic musculoskeletal radiographs transmitted by electronic mail. *Journal of Orthopaedic Trauma* 13(7):516–519.

Ricci MA, Caputo M, Amour J, Rogers FB, Sartorelli K, Callas PW, Malone PT. 2003. Telemedicine reduces discrepancies in rural trauma care. *Telemedicine Journal and e-Health* 9(1):3-11.

Richwine M, McGowan JJ. 2001. A rural virtual health sciences library project: Research findings with implications for next generation library services. *Bulletin of the Medical Library Association* 89(1):37–44.

Romano MJ, Hernandez J, Gaylor A, Howard S, Knox R. 2001. Improvement in asthma symptoms and quality of life in pediatric patients through specialty care delivered via telemedicine. *Telemedicine Journal and e-Health* 7(4):281–286.

Rosenblatt R. 2000. The health of rural people and the communities and environments in which they live. In: Geyman JP, Norris TE, Hart GL, eds. *Textbook of Rural Medicine.* New York: McGraw-Hill. Pp. 3–14.

Rosenfeld BA, Dorman T, Breslow MJ, Pronovost P, Jenckes M, Zhang N, Anderson G, Rubin H. 2000. Intensive care unit telemedicine: Alternate paradigm for providing continuous interventist care. *Critical Care Medicine* 28(12):3925–3931.

Rotvold GH, Knarvik U, Johansen MA, Fossen K. 2003. Telemedicine screening for diabetic retinopathy: Staff and patient satisfaction. *Journal of Telemedicine and Telecare* 9(2):109–113.

Rundle RL. 2002 (June 25). Healthcare providers let patients view records online. *The Wall Street Journal.* P. B1.

RUS (Rural Utilities Service). 2004. *RUS Rural Broadband Loan and Loan Guarantee Program.* [Online]. Available: http://www.usda.gov/rus/telecom/broadband.htm [accessed June 30, 2004].

Sable C. 2001. Telecardiology: A potential impact on acute care. *Critical Care Medicine* 29(8 Supplement):N159–N165.

Sanders J, Brucker P, Miller MD. 1995. Using telemedicine for continuing education for rural physicians. *Academic Medicine* 70(5):457.

Sittig DF, Kuperman GJ, Fiskio J. 1999. *Evaluating Physician Satisfaction Regarding User Interactions with an Electronic Medical Record System.* Paper presented at the meeting of the Proceedings of Annual American Medical Informatics Association Symposium. Bethesda, MD: American Medical Informatics Association.

Smith CE, Cha JJ, Kleinbeck SV, Clements SA, Cook D, Koehler J. 2002. Feasibility of in-home telehealth form conducting nursing research. *Clinical Nursing Research* 11(2):220–233.

Smithline N, Christenson E. 2001. Physicians and the Internet: Understanding where we are and where we are going. *Journal of Ambulatory Care Management* 24(4):39–53.

Spatz M. 2000. Providing consumer health information in the rural setting: Planetree health resources center's approach. *Bulletin of the Medical Library Association* 88(4):382–388.

Stanberry B. 2000. Telemedicine: Barriers and opportunities in the 21st century. *Journal of Internal Medicine* 247(6):615–628.

Strode CA, Rubal BJ, Gerhardt RT, Bulgrin JR, Boyd SR. 2003. Wireless and satellite transmission of prehospital focused abdominal sonography for trauma. *Prehospital Emergency Care* 7(3):375–379.

Taylor H, Leitman R. 2001. *New Data Show Internet, Website and E-Mail Usage by Physicians All Increasing.* HarrisInteractive. [Online]. Available: http://www.harrisinteractive.com/news/newsletters/healthnews/HI_HealthCareNews2001Vol1_iss8.pdf [accessed May 5, 2004].

Tierney WM. 2001. Improving clinical decisions and outcomes with information: A review. *International Journal of Medical Informatics* 62(1):1–9.

Trippi JA, Kopp G, Lee KS, Morrison H, Risk G, Jones JH, Cordell WH, Chrapla M, Nelson D. 1996. The feasibility of dobutamine stress echocardiography in the emergency department with telemedicine interpretation. *Journal of the American Society of Echocardiography* 9(2):113–118.

USAC (Universal Service Administrative Company). 2004. *About RHCD.* [Online]. Available: http://www.rhc.universalservice.org/overview/rhcd.asp [accessed September 14, 2004].

Varon J, Marik PE. 2002. Clinical information systems and the electronic medical record in the intensive care unit. *Current Opinion in Critical Care* 8(6):616–624.

Versweyveld, L. 2001. *High Plains Rural Health Network Starts Using e-Ceptionist Scheduling Service.* [Online]. Available: http://www.hoise.com/vmw/02/articles/vmw/LV-VM-01-02-3.html [accessed July 7, 2004].

Von Knoop C, Lovich D, Silverstein MB, Tutty M. 2003. *Vital Signs: e-Health in the United States.* Boston, MA: The Boston Consulting Group.

Waegemann CP. 2002. *Status Report 2002: Electronic Health Records*. [Online]. Available: http://www.medrecinst.com/uploadedFiles/MRILibrary/StatusReport.pdf [accessed May 5, 2004].

Wakefield M. 2002. Patient safety and medical errors: Implications for rural health care. *Journal of Legal Medicine* 23:43–56.

Wallingford KT, Ruffin AB, Ginter KA, Spann ML, Johnson FE, Dutcher GA, Mehnert R, Nash DL, Bridgers JW, Lyon BJ, Siegel ER, Roderer NK. 1996. Outreach activities of the NLM: A five-year review. *Bulletin of the Medical Library Association* 84(2 Supplement):1–60.

Wellever, A. 1999. *Organizing for Achievement: Three Rural Health Network Case Studies*. [Online]. Available: http://ruralhealth.hrsa.gov/pub/organizing.htm [accessed June 2004].

WH (The White House). 2004a. *Promoting Innovation and Competitiveness*. [Online]. Available: http://www.whitehouse.gov/infocus/technology/economic_policy 200404/chap3.html [accessed June 14, 2004].

WH. 2004b. *A New Generation of American Innovation*. [Online]. Available: http:// www.whitehouse.gov/infocus/technology/economic_policy200404/innovation.pdf [accessed July 25, 2004].

WH. 2004c. *Executive Order #13335*. [Online]. Available: http://www.whitehouse.gov/ news/releases/2004/04/20040427-4.html [accessed May 2004].

White M, Dorman SM. 2001. Receiving social support online: Implications for health education. *Health Education Research* 16(6):693–707.

Wholey D, Moscovice I, Hietpas T, Hotzman J. 2003. *The Environmental Context of Patient Safety and Medical Errors*. [Online]. Available: http://www.hsr.umn.edu/ rhrc/pdfs/wpaper/working%20paper%20047.pdf [accessed March 2004].

Wood FB, Sahali R, Press N, Burroughs C, Mala TA, Siegel ER, Rambo N, Fuller SS. 2003. Tribal connections health information outreach: Results, evaluation, and challenges. *Journal of the Medical Library Association* 91(1):57–66.

Yellowlees P. 1997. Successful development of telemedicine systems: Seven core principles. *Journal of Telemedicine and Telecare* 3(4):215–222.

Appendixes

A

Biographies of Committee Members

Mary Wakefield, Ph.D., R.N., F.A.A.N., Chair, is Director and Professor, Center for Rural Health at the University of North Dakota School of Medicine and Health Sciences in Grand Forks, North Dakota; and Adjunct Professor at the University of North Dakota College of Nursing. Previously she was Professor and Director, Center for Health Policy, at George Mason University, Fairfax, Virginia. In the 1990s, she served in staff positions in the U.S. Senate, culminating with the position of Chief of Staff to Senator Kent Conrad. Throughout her tenure on Capitol Hill, Dr. Wakefield advised on a range of public health policy issues, drafted legislative proposals, and worked with interest groups and other Senate offices. She cochaired the Senate Rural Health Caucus Staff Organization. In this capacity, she was directly involved with a wide range of rural health policy issues, including recruitment and retention of health care providers, reimbursement, emergency services, and telemedicine, among others. Dr. Wakefield's major research interests and expertise encompass the quality of rural health care, Native American health issues, the rural workforce, rural emergency medical services, rural patient safety, and Medicare payment policies and related impacts on rural providers. She has served on many advisory and expert committees, including MEDPAC; the National Advisory Committee on Rural Health, Department of Health and Human Services (DHHS); and committees of the IOM. She is a member of the Institute of Medicine (IOM) Board on Health Care Services.

Calvin Beale, M.S., is Senior Demographer, Economic Research Service, U.S. Department of Agriculture. His research has focused on topics related to the populations of rural and small-town America, including race and ethnic composition, distribution, migration, poverty, and growth and decline, as well as the implications of trends for public policy. He has written more than 100 articles and reports on demographic subjects. He is also author of a book of collected writings—*A Taste of the Country*—edited by Peter Morrison (1990), and coauthor of two books, *Rural and Small Town America* (1989) and *Economic Areas of the United States* (1961). In 2002, he was honored by the Rural Sociological Society and the Annie Casey Foundation for his work in the field of rural demography.

Andrew Coburn, Ph.D., is Professor of Health Policy and Management, Director of the Institute for Health Policy, and Associate Dean at the Muskie School of Public Service, University of Southern Maine. Dr. Coburn's research has addressed the problems of rural health care delivery and financing, health insurance and the uninsured, and Medicaid policy. In the early 1990s he established the Maine Rural Health Research Center, which has focused on rural health insurance coverage, behavioral health, rural hospitals, and long-term care issues. His research addresses problems of rural health care financing and delivery, including rural quality and patient safety, health insurance coverage, and rural hospitals. His recent research includes studies of rural hospital patient safety, the impact of the Medicare Rural Hospital Flexibility program, and patterns of health coverage for rural populations. Dr. Coburn has published widely on these topics and has testified often before Congress on the rural impacts of federal policy changes. He currently serves on the Rural Policy Research Institute's Expert Panel on Rural Health Delivery. He has been an active member of Academy Health and the National Academy for State Health Policy. He received the National Rural Health Association's Distinguished Researcher Award in 2001.

Don E. Detmer, M.D., M.A., is Professor Emeritus and Professor of Medical Education, Department of Health Evaluation Sciences, University of Virginia, and Senior Associate, Judge Institute of Management, University of Cambridge. He is Vice Chair of the China Medical Board of New York, Inc., Chair of Section 12 of the membership committee of the IOM, a Trustee of the Nuffield Trust of London, Cochair of the Blue Ridge Group, Research Director of the J&J Centre for Advancing Health Information, and Chair of the International Committee of the American Medical Informatics Association. He is a lifetime Associate of the National Academies and a fellow of the American Association for the Advancement of Science, Academy Health, and the American Colleges of Medical Informatics, Surgeons, and Sports Medicine. From 1999 to 2003, he was Dennis Gillings Professor of Health Management and Director, Cambridge University Health, the health policy center at the Judge Institute of Management, Cambridge's business school. Prior to his years in England, he was Vice President for Health Sciences at the Universities of Virginia and Utah and on the faculty at the University of Wisconsin-Madison. He is immediate past Chairman of the Board on Health Care Services of the IOM and the National Committee on Vital and Health Statistics and has also chaired the Board of Regents of the National Library of Medicine. His education included a medical degree from the University of Kansas and subsequent training at the National Institutes of Health, the Johns Hopkins Hospital, Duke University Medical Center, the IOM, and Harvard Business School. His masters degree is from the University of Cambridge. Dr. Detmer's career includes innovative work in national health information policy, quality improvement, administrative medicine, vascular surgery, sports medicine, and masters-level education programs for clinician-executives.

Jim Grigsby, Ph.D., is Associate Professor, University of Colorado Health Sciences Center (UCHSC), in Denver, Colorado, and Associate Director of the Center for Health Services Research at UCHSC. Since 1993 he has studied different aspects of telemedicine, especially implemention in rural settings. His most recent work on telehealth has focused on the diffusion of technology in home health care and in chronic disease management. His current research includes medication errors during inpatient–outpatient care transitions, the effectiveness of telemedicine, telemedicine payment policy, telehealth and rural mental health, effects of cognitive impairment on the effectiveness of chronic disease self-management in older adults, effects on cognition of cancer chemotherapy, and the characterization of clinical and neuroradiological features of a novel neurodegenerative disorder affecting older male carriers of Fragile X syndrome. Dr. Grisby has worked closely with rural telemedicine providers and researchers in Iowa, North Carolina, and Nebraska, and was involved in the development of a project to assess the suitability of telehealth technology for critical access hospitals in Wisconsin. He has published extensively in peer-reviewed journals; authored chapters in books, technical reports, and monographs; and written letters in scientific journals on telemedicine and on the use of simulated neural networks to predict risk-adjusted medical outcomes. Dr. Grigsby is on the editorial board of the *Telemedicine Journal and e-Health* and served on the Technical Advisory Panel to the IOM Committee on Telemedicine.

David Hartley, Ph.D., M.H.A., is Director, Division of Rural Health, Muskie School of Public Service, at the University of Southern Maine, Portland. His current research is focused on rural mental health services, the mental health workforce, the rural safety net, rural hospital scope of services, and a national evaluation of the Medicare Rural Hospital Flexibility Program. His doctorate is in health services research, policy and administration, and biomedical ethics. He has published many reports, monographs, and articles, several of which address issues of rural mental and behavioral health, rural health networks, and the rural safety net. He has presented papers at meetings of Academy Health, the National Conference of State Mental Health Program Directors, and the National Rural Health Association, as well as regional meetings of the National Association of State Offices of Rural Health and the New England and Maine Rural Health Associations. He also sits on the National Rural Health Association's Rural Health Policy Board. Dr. Hartley received the National Rural Health Association's Distinguished Researcher Award in 2003.

Sandral Hullett, M.D., M.P.H., is CEO of Jefferson Health System/Cooper Green Hospital in Birmingham, Alabama. She was formerly Executive Director of Family HealthCare of America, a not-for-profit community health center serving 40 rural counties throughout Alabama. Her interests include rural health care and health care planning and delivery of care to the underserved, underinusured, and poor. She was awarded the University of Alabama School of Public Health's first Public Health Hero Award for her work in providing compassionate care to people living in Alabama's rural, impoverished Black Belt communities. Dr. Hullett is a member of the IOM and has served on several IOM committees, including the Committee on the Changing Market, Managed Care, and Future Viability of Safety Net Providers. Dr. Hullett received her M.D. from the Medical College of Pennsylvania and her M.P.H. from the University of Alabama.

A. Clinton MacKinney, M.D., M.S., is a Senior Consultant with Stroudwater Associates, assisting rural hospitals in implementing performance improvements. In addition, he works as a rural emergency department physician in Little Falls, Minnesota, and as a health services researcher with the Rural

Policy and Research Institute (RUPRI) Research Center, Nebraska Medical Center. Until recently, he served as Medical Director for Health Partners Central Minnesota Clinics in St. Cloud, Minnesota. Prior to assuming that position, he practiced family medicine for 14 years in a rural Iowa community of 4,000. Dr. MacKinney's experience and research interests include geriatrics, chronic disease management, hospital/physician relationships, community health systems development, rural health quality, and rural health policy. He is a member of the RUPRI Health Panel and serves on several boards of nonprofit organizations, such as the Roundhouse Group and the Minnesota Center for Rural Health. Dr. MacKinney has lectured and published on rural health, and has served on committees for the American Medical Association, the American Academy of Family Physicians, The Robert Wood Johnson Foundation, and the National Rural Health Association.

Ira Moscovice, Ph.D., is Professor, Division of Health Services Research and Policy, at the University of Minnesota. He is director of the Rural Health Research Center at the University of Minnesota and has written extensively on issues related to rural health care and the use of health services research to improve health policy decision making in state government. Dr. Moscovice was the first recipient of the National Rural Health Association's Distinguished Researcher Award in 1992. In 2002, he received a Robert Wood Johnson Foundation Investigator Award in Health Policy Research. He has served as principal investigator for numerous rural health studies funded by, among others, the Federal Office of Rural Health Policy, the Centers for Medicare and Medicaid Services, the Agency for Healthcare Research and Quality (AHRQ), The Robert Wood Johnson Foundation, and the Northwest Area Foundation. His current research interests include the implementation and assessment of rural health networks and managed care, the evaluation of alternative rural health care delivery systems, and the quality of rural health care. Dr. Moscovice currently serves on the Health Services Research Study Section of AHRQ and the National Advisory Committee of the Coming Home Program of The Robert Wood Johnson Foundation, and previously served on the IOM's Access to Health Care Services Monitoring Committee.

Roger Rosenblatt, M.D., M.P.H., M.F.R., is Professor and Vice Chair, Department of Family Medicine, and Adjunct Professor, Department of Health Services, School of Public Health and Community Medicine, at the University of Washington. He is founder and co-Principal Investigator of the Rural

Health Research Center at the University of Washington. He has done extensive research in the delivery of health services to rural populations in the United States and around the world. He is particularly interested in improving the supply and the quality of health services in isolated and sparsely populated areas, and has published widely on these issues. He has worked as a Medical Officer and a Regional Program Director for the National Health Service Corps of the United States Public Health Service, has been a consultant to a number of governmental agencies that deal with rural health services, and has testified before Congress on these issues. He is a member of several associations and organizations, including the American Public Health Association, Academy Health, the National Rural Health Association, the Region X Rural Health Coordinating Committee, and the Rural Hospital Facilities Task Force.

Tim Size, M.B.A, B.S.E., has been Executive Director of the 29-hospital Rural Wisconsin Health Cooperative since helping to found it in 1979 while working as an administrator at the University of Wisconsin Hospital and Clinics. He helped start HMO of Wisconsin in 1984, leading to varied experience with rural managed care. He represents a rural health perspective on numerous boards and commissions within Wisconsin. He is past President of the National Rural Health Association and served as a member of then DHHS Secretary Donna Shalala's National Advisory Committee on Rural Health. He is currently serving on DHHS Secretary Tommy Thompson's National Advisory Committee on Rural Health and Human Services. He was a Kellogg National Fellow and has received the National Rural Health Association's Louis Gorin Award for Outstanding Achievement in Rural Health Care. He lays claim to the only monthly cartoon series in the country focused on rural health.

Linda Watson, M.L.S., is Associate Dean and Director, Claude Moore Health Sciences Library, University of Virginia, and Lecturer in the School of Medicine's Department of Health Evaluation Sciences. She was President of the Medical Library Association in 2002–2003 and currently serves on the National Institutes of Health's PubMed Central National Advisory Committee. Her prior experience includes 10 years at the National Library of Medicine, where she held various management positions, specializing in nonprint media. She has published and made many presentations in her field. She has managed several grant projects, including, among others, establishment of a partnership between the University of Virginia and the Danville Regional

Medical Center for improving information access in rural south-central Virginia, and Grateful Med Outreach to rural nurses and physicians in Virginia. She has developed programs for the rural outreach of medical information into the far corners of southwest Virginia for both health professionals and citizens, and has recently worked with the Hispanic migrant population in the rural Shenandoah Valley of Virginia.

B

Characteristics of Rural Populations[1]

Rural America encompasses a wide range of regional differences. Over the last 50 years, many rural areas have become more densely settled by acquiring new residents and sources of employment, or suburbanized by increases in commuting to jobs in urban areas. Other regions remain stagnant or in steady decline, having been unable to transition from what was once a largely agricultural settlement. Finally, some are simply more remote and less populated. Degree of rurality versus urbanization is defined on a continuum.

DEFINING RURAL AMERICA

In general, a rural area is considered a place of low population density. The three most common definitions of rural areas are provided by the Department of Commerce, Bureau of the Census; the White House Office of Management and Budget (OMB); and the Department of Agriculture (USDA) Economic Research Service (ERS). Table B-1 provides an overview of each agency's methodology.

---

[1] Some sections of this appendix were adapted from a commissioned paper by Calvin L. Beale and John B. Cromartie entitled "Profile of the Rural Population" (February 24, 2004).

The Census Bureau has the longest-standing definition of rural as open country and settlements of less than 2,500 residents, excluding suburbs of urbanized areas with 50,000 or more population. For the 2000 census, revised tabulating procedures extended the classification of urban-like suburbs to include small towns ("urbanized areas").[2] This transferred a number of people to urban status who had previously been classified as rural, especially in the Northeast. In 2000, the rural population was measured at 59.0 million, or 21 percent of the total population.

OMB expands the Census Bureau's definition to a county-based approach to measure the extent to which a large city's (central city) economic influence extends beyond its limits. The level of intercounty job commuting is the principal means of determination. The terms "metropolitan," "micropolitan," and "noncore" are used to describe the areas of measurement. A metropolitan area is defined as a county with a central city and its adjoining counties that together have more than 50,000 people, regardless of the size of the largest central city (FR, 2000). Micropolitan areas are defined as counties that have a town of at least 10,000 population; outlying counties are included if commuting to the central county is 25 percent or higher. Noncore counties are those not near an urbanized area of 10,000 or more. Most recently, the 2004 Omnibus Appropriations Bill broadened the definition of rural to include any incorporated city or town of 20,000 persons or less rather than using the OMB definition in order to broaden eligibility for participation in USDA's Rural Broadband Grant and Loan Program.

The ERS has developed two other types of measurements for population comparisons—the rural–urban continuum codes and the urban influence codes. The rural–urban continuum codes (see Figure B-1) are used to distinguish metropolitan counties by size and nonmetropolitan counties by their degree of urbanization and adjacency to metropolitan areas. Metropolitan areas can measure more than 1 million or less than 250,000, and nonmetropolitan codes range from +20,000, adjacent to a metropolitan area, to completely rural, or <2,500 not adjacent.

---

[2] Free-standing towns of 2,500 to 9,999 are often considered rural because of their modest scale and relevance to providing health services for a larger surrounding rural area; counting these towns would add another 11.1 million to the rural total. Above this, 7.6 million live in clusters of 10,000 to 19,999 population, and 11.3 million in clusters of 20,000 to 49,999. The population total of all the rural and urban cluster categories is 89 million (FR, 2000).

TABLE B-1 Methodologies Used to Define Rural Areas

	Bureau of the Census Population Density	OMB Metropolitan, Micropolitan,[a] and Noncore[b] Statistical Areas
Methodology	Population density measured in units smaller than the county level.	Metropolitan and micropolitan areas measured at the county level.
Application	More detailed measurement and analysis of the local community.	Assesses the extent to which a large city's economic influence extends beyond its limit.
Urban/Metro Definition	Urbanized areas (UAs) include a central city and surrounding densely settled areas of at least 2,500 population that together have a population of 50,000 or more and a population density exceeding 1,000 per square mile. Urban clusters include free-standing towns of 20,000–49,000, 10,000–19,000, 2,500–9,999. Definitions applied in year 2000.	Core-based statistical areas (CBSAs) include metropolitan and micropolitan areas. Each metropolitan CBSA must have at least one UA of 50,000 population or more. Micropolitan CBSAs must have at least one urban cluster of 10,000–49,999. Nonmetropolitan areas can include micropolitan areas and noncore areas (what is thought of as rural). Definitions applied in year 2000.
IOM Determinations of Rural for This Report	Rural areas are considered those with 2,500 or less population.	Noncore nonmetropolitan areas outside metropolitan CBSAs.

Economic Research Service Rural–Urban Continuum Codes	Economic Research Service Urban Influence Codes
Rural–urban continuum codes measured by county.	County-based measurements that are more subdivided than the continuum codes.
Evaluates urbanization and adjacency to metro areas using a nine-tiered system.	Evaluates status according to micropolitan and noncore status using a 12-tiered system.

Metro counties
–counties in metro areas of 1 million or more,
–counties in metro areas of 250,000–1 million, and
–counties in metro areas of fewer than 250,000.

Nonmetropolitan counties
–urban population of 20,000+, adjacent to metro area,
–urban population of 20,000+, not adjacent to metro area,
–urban population of 2,500–19,999, adjacent to metro area,
–urban population of 2,500–19,999, not adjacent to metro area,
–completely rural or less than 2,500 urban population, adjacent to metro area, and
–completely rural or less than 2,500, not adjacent to metro area.
Definitions applied in year 2003.

Metro counties
–counties in large metro area of 1 million or more, and
–counties in small metro areas of <1 million.

Nonmetropolitan counties
–micropolitan counties adjacent to large metro areas,
–noncore counties adjacent to large metro areas,
–micropolitan counties adjacent to small metro areas,
–noncore counties adjacent to small metro areas,
–noncore counties adjacent to small metro areas with own town,
–micropolitan counties not adjacent to a metro area,
–noncore counties adjacent to a micropolitan area with own town,
–noncore counties adjacent to a micropolitan area with no own town, or micropolitan area with own town, and
–noncore counties not adjacent to a metro or micropolitan area with no own town.
Definitions applied in year 2003.

Can be considered codes 8 and 9.

Can be considered codes 11 and 12.

continued

TABLE B-1   Continued

	Bureau of the Census Population Density	OMB Metropolitan, Micropolitan,[a] and Noncore[b] Statistical Areas
Rural Population Percentages	Rural population = 59 million, 21 percent of total population.	Noncore nonmetropolitan population = 22.1 million, 8 percent of total population.
Frontier Population	Not applicable	Not applicable

[a] Micropolitan is defined using OMB's designation of urban clusters (counties that have a town of at least 10,000). Outlying counties are included if commuting to the central county is 25 percent or higher. Any nonmetropolitan area with an urban cluster becomes the central county of a micropolitan area.
[b] Noncore counties are not near an urban cluster of 10,000 or more.

"Frontier areas," a term used mainly by rural health and agriculture officials, are considered the most thinly settled counties, with population densities of fewer than seven households per square mile. Figure B-2 provides an overview of frontier areas. About 383 counties have frontier-level density and are near a small metropolitan area or cluster of 10,000–49,999.

POPULATION CHANGE

During the period of economic prosperity from 1990 to 2000, 30 percent of all nonmetropolitan counties experienced population growth of 13.1 percent or more (Beale and Cromartie, 2004). The growth was due to two dynamics: (1) increases in commuting to jobs in suburban/urban/metro areas by many long-term rural residents in terms of both frequency and distance of commutes; and (2) increases in the numbers of urban residents moving to the country and small-town locations to have lower housing costs or to live in less congestion. While population growth generally strengthens the local economy, it also increases demand for health services. As discussed in other parts of this report, most rural areas lack an adequate health care

Economic Research Service Rural–Urban Continuum Codes	Economic Research Service Urban Influence Codes
Nonmetropolitan rural population (codes 8 and 9) = 5.2 million, 1.8 percent of total population.	Nonmetropolitan rural population (codes 11 and 12) = 3.2 million, 8.1 percent of total population.

Although the rural–urban continuum codes and urban influence codes do not include parameters for frontier areas, the USDA ERS uses the following definition for measurements: frontier areas = 7 households per square mile.

Frontier population = 2.9 million,[c] 1.0 percent of total population.

[c] Calculations are based on the county's average density per square mile, and in some cases the county may contain a small town. Methods for measuring solely those living in frontier areas of <7 households per square mile (rather than averages of county statistics) are being developed at this time. SOURCE: ERS, 2003a; FR, 2000.

infrastructure to meet the needs of their current population, let alone their projected future population assuming current growth trends continue.

A significant geographic trend is the decline in population in nonmetropolitan counties of the Great Plains from the Canadian border to south Texas, with a continuing high dependence on agriculture. These areas have experienced prolonged outmigration of young adults, resulting in higher proportions of older people and increasing problems with access to medical services. About 313 counties have no urban settlement of 10,000 or more and are not adjacent to a county having such a place. The population density averages 4.2 persons per square mile. These residents experience the core of the rural medical access problems related to scale of settlement discussed in this report. Some hospitals and pharmacies have closed, and residents are more distant from physicians, with less choice of providers.

Persistent decline is also found in parts of the lower South where there is a significant population of African Americans or there has been a major drop in coal mining jobs. The populations in parts of the Allegheny and Cumberland Plateaus have declined as well because of sustained losses in the manufacturing sector.

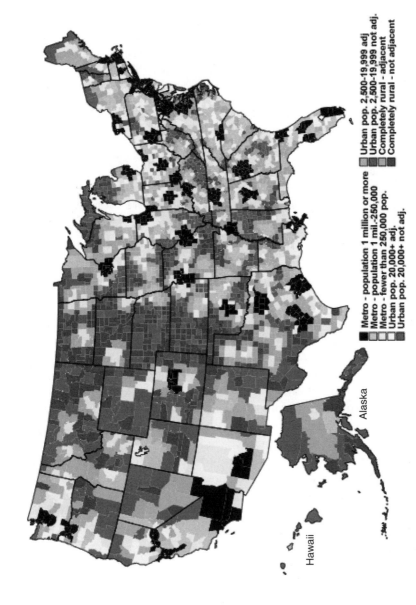

FIGURE B-1 USDA Economic Research Service: Rural–urban continuum code classifications.
SOURCE: ERS, 2003a.

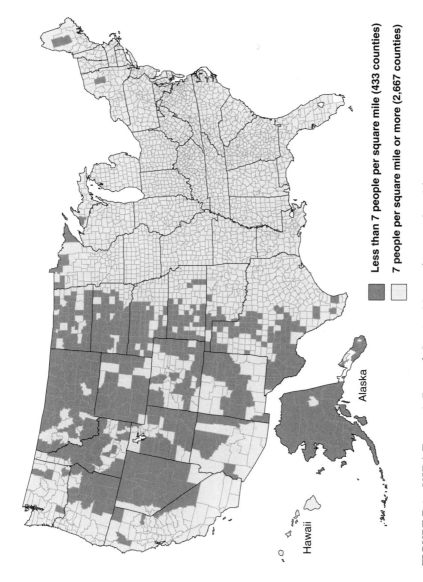

FIGURE B-2 USDA Economic Research Service: Metropolitan, rural, and frontier areas.
SOURCE: Beale and Cromartie, 2004.

Less than 7 people per square mile (433 counties)

7 people per square mile or more (2,667 counties)

Alaska

Hawaii

AGE DISTRIBUTION

The age distribution and level of rurality of a county influence the health status and health care needs of its population (Gamm et al., 2002; NCHS, 2001). Since the 1960s, the age structure of the population in a geographic area has tended to become older as urbanization has decreased (Beale and Cromartie, 2004; CMS, 2004). This upward urban–rural gradient for those aged 65+ is present in all regions (but steepest in the Midwest and South) and is due to changes in migration patterns—that is, retired persons migrating *into* rural areas, coupled with a half-century of younger persons migrating *out* of rural areas.[3] According to the ERS, 315 rural counties experienced a rise in their older population (aged 60+) by 15 percent or more as a result of net migration alone during the 1990s (NCHS, 2001). By 2000, this amounted to 24+ percent of the population seeking rural counties as retirement destinations (see Figure B-3). Aside from migration, the overall growth in the older population from 1990 to 2000 was 7.4 percent (Personal communication, C. Beale, June 1, 2004). The growth rate of the older rural population is expected to be quite high over the next 20 years as the baby boomers move into retirement age.[4]

This increasing age trend has significant implications for health care needs. As noted in this report, older people have a higher incidence of chronic conditions, and many have multiple such conditions (Anderson and Horvath, 2002). Residents in rural areas experience higher rates of limitations in daily activities[5] as a result of their chronic conditions—activity limitation levels are about 20 percent in rural individuals compared with 13 percent for their urban counterparts (NCHS, 2001). Effective management of chronic conditions requires ongoing access to a multidisciplinary team of providers, including primary care providers, specialists, pharmacists, health educators, and social workers. As discussed in Chapter 4, many rural communities struggle to attract and retain an adequate health professions workforce to meet the needs of their population.

---

[3] In particular, the large older populations of the Plains and the Corn Belt reflect the prolonged outbound movement of young people to urban areas over more than a generation.

[4] Nationally, the population of those aged 60+ is expected to grow by 23 percent from 2000 to 2010, and then by 33 percent from 2010 to 2020—far higher than the growth rate of the rest of the population (Personal communication, C. Beale, June 1, 2004).

[5] Activities reflected in this measure may include, but are not limited to, working independently performing routine tasks such as household chores or shopping, and independently performing personal care activities such as bathing or eating (NCHS, 2001).

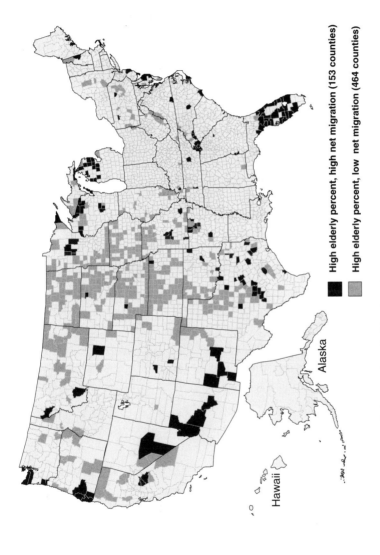

FIGURE B-3 USDA Economic Research Service: Rural older Americans.

NOTE: High elderly percent = 24 percent or more of the population aged 60 or older, 2000; high net migration = 15 percent growth from net migration of the population aged 60 or older, 1990–2000.

SOURCE: Beale and Cromartie, 2004.

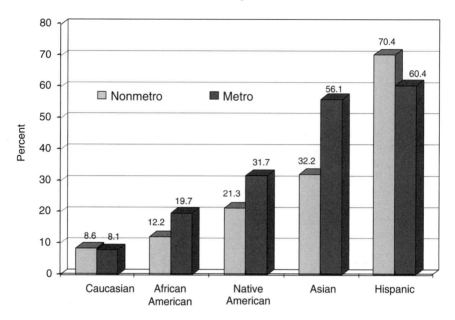

FIGURE B-4 USDA Economic Research Service: Population grouth rates by race and ethnicity, nonmetro and metro areas, 1990–2000.
SOURCE: Compiled by ERS from 1990 and 2000 Census data, U.S. Census Bureau.

Although the overall trend in most rural communities has been toward a higher age distribution, certain rural areas did experience a rebound of younger people in the 1990s (PRB, 1999). This may mean that raising families in these areas has growing appeal. Rural communities experiencing these trends will need to ensure an adequate supply of primary care, obstetric, pediatric, and emergency services.

RACIAL AND ETHNIC TRENDS

Minority groups are also a growing proportion of rural and small town populations, particularly among children and younger, working-age adults. Figure B-4 provides an overview of the population growth rates by race and ethnicity in metropolitan and rural areas from 1990 to 2000. For the 2000 census, 10.2 million rural residents identified themselves as belonging to racial or ethnic groups—a 30 percent increase over the last decade (Census, 2003b). In particular, 16 percent belong to one of three primary groups—African American, American Indian/Alaska Native, or Hispanic—while 2 percent belong to the Asian/Hawaiian/Pacific Islander group or some other group, or consider themselves multiracial. Of the primary groups, 43 percent live in 356 counties where they constitute one-third or more of the population.

African Americans are well distributed across the South's lowland districts from southern Maryland through Louisiana. Although the 1990s brought gains in education and income, many difficulties persist for African American residents, who are predominately lower-income (e.g., lack of transportation, lack of affordable health care, poor housing). Native Americans are clustered in the northern High Plains, the Four Corners region in the Southwest, and Alaska. Counties in the first two regions contain reservations on which Native Americans are exercising greater economic and political control; however, poverty and unemployment remain high. For Alaska Natives, low population density and isolation from major population centers severely limit economic development prospects and increase health care delivery costs. High population concentrations of rural Hispanics remain in counties along the Rio Grande Valley, from the headwaters in southern Colorado to the Gulf of Mexico; however, about 50 percent now live outside the Southwest. Growing geographic dispersion has increased rural racial/ethnic diversity in all regions, particularly the Midwest and Southeast.

Generally, rural counties with high minority populations show signs of economic disadvantage. Minorities often live in isolated communities or neighborhoods where poverty is high, opportunity is low, and economic benefits from education and training are limited. Many who acquire education or technical skills must apply them elsewhere. Because of their socioeconomic status, minority groups tend to rely heavily on safety net services supported by federal and state programs, and resources for these programs are often inadequate (Rosenblatt, 2000).

While minority groups have many commonalities, some groups have distinct health care needs. By the end of the 1990s, Hispanics accounted for over 25 percent of the population growth in rural counties, with their population ranging from 8 percent in the Midwest to 18–29 percent in other rural regions (ERS, 2004). A large percentage of rural Hispanics work in agriculture as relatively low-paid, seasonal or part-time farm laborers, and many are uninsured (Ricketts, 1999). Hispanics also tend to have higher fertility levels, lower median ages, and larger household sizes (with more children and fewer elderly) (Beale and Cromartie, 2004). Rural communities with large populations of Hispanics need to ensure the availability of safety net programs that provide primary care and obstetric and pediatric services, and can address language and literacy barriers.

INCOME AND EMPLOYMENT

Income level and type of employment determine socioeconomic status and have a significant influence on the health status of rural residents. The predominance of lower-wage jobs, limited availability of year-round work, and less education in rural regions leave individuals and communities at an economic disadvantage, and frequently without health insurance or income to spend on health care. Thus, they are less likely to receive the health care they need to prevent and/or manage health conditions. The result is poorer outcomes and often higher long-term health care expenditures (IOM, 2002).

Rural areas are falling behind in the new economy. Job growth in rural counties fell below that in urban areas in 1995 and has been substantially lower (at 1 percent) ever since (Zhang and Bowman, 1998). Today, only a small portion of the rural population, 5.7 percent, is directly employed in agriculture—once the livelihood of rural America. Industries that are important to the rural economy include the public sector, supplying 22 percent of earnings; consumer services (e.g., retail and personal services, private health and education services), also supplying 22 percent; manufacturing at 19 percent; and producer services (related to agriculture and fisheries) at 11.5 percent (ERS, 2003c). Bureau of Economic Analysis data also indicate significant growth in the finance, insurance, and real estate sector and the construction sector (ERS, 2002). As of third quarter 2003, the seasonally adjusted unemployment rate for rural areas was 6 percent—a rate that urban areas have reached with unemployment rising regularly since 2000 (ERS, 2003a).

Estimates of the median nonmetropolitan household income from 1996 to 2001 average $34,135, nearly one-fourth below the average for metro areas of $45,938 (Census, 2003a).[6] For the same period, the poverty rate grew by 20 percent over that in the 1990s in 444 nonmetropolitan counties[7] (e.g., the poverty rate is annual income <$16,895 for a family of two adults and two minor children).[8] In 2000, a total of 494 counties had poverty levels of

---

[6] Weekly earnings for nonmetropolitan residents who had completed high school (but no further training) averaged $458, just 59 percent of the $782 weekly average earned by college graduates. Some of this difference may be offset by lower costs of living in rural areas (e.g., housing, local taxes); however, the variation is not substantial enough to be meaningful.

[7] Fully 93 percent of these counties are areas with high populations of African Americans, Hispanics, Native Americans, or non-Hispanic Caucasians of the Southern Highlands. The population typically has lower-than-average educational attainment, a lower percentage of persons working or having year-round full-time work, a higher proportion of children living in a female-headed family with no husband present, and higher frequency of persons with a disability.

[8] Using 2000 data, 14.6 percent of rural (and 11.8 percent of metro) populations had household incomes below the poverty threshold used by the federal government.

20 percent or more; of these, 422 were in rural areas and 72 in urban. Consistent poverty over four consecutive censuses from 1970 to 2000 was most prevalent in 386 counties—340 in rural areas and 46 in urban (Personal communication, C. Beale, June 2, 2004). For both urban and rural areas, the most extensive poverty was among 43 percent of female-headed single-parent households with children under 18. Poverty was less frequent among older adults (13 percent) than among children (17 percent).

Lower-income individuals consistently have a higher incidence of health problems. Among families earning less than $20,000 in income in 2001, 25 percent reported some limitation in "usual activities" stemming from health problems, compared with just 6.3 percent among persons in families with more than $55,000 in income (NCHS, 2001). Because the demographics of income and employment have close ties to the demographics of ethnic and racial groups, individuals in these conditions are similarly and disproportionately dependent on publicly provided health care safety net services.

Even lower-income individuals who are working often lack health insurance (IOM, 2004). As the cost of health insurance continues to increase, more and more employers, especially small and medium-sized ones, choose to provide no or only minimal health insurance benefits to their employees. Methods must be found to assist small and medium-sized employers in obtaining affordable health insurance. In addition, employers need to become more engaged in providing their employees with resources for health/wellness education and disease management programs, perhaps through partnerships with other local community organizations to share resources.

EDUCATION AND LITERACY

Sizable gains in higher levels of education are being realized in rural areas: 77 percent of rural residents have graduated high school or acquired a General Educational Development (GED) credential,[9] and rural school children are performing about as well as county central city children on standardized tests (Ricketts, 1999); however, both rural and central city children still lag behind suburban children on most indicators. Rural schools have some advantages—smaller sizes; more cooperative relationships among teachers, parents, and community organizations; and lower student–teacher

---

[9] In 2000, only 23 percent of rural adults had not graduated from high school or acquired a GED credential, as compared with 31 percent in 1990, a shift to a proportion closer to that of urban adults at 18 percent (ERS, 2003b).

ratios. However, they also have several disadvantages—fewer advanced course offerings, less attention to college preparation, lower college graduation rates, inadequate physical and educational resources, and higher dropout rates (Marshall, 2004).

Weaknesses in the school curriculum have been an impediment to attracting families with young children to move to or remain in rural communities despite the lower cost of living. Rural high schools offer fewer vocational educational programs than their nonrural counterparts. Rural schools focus on common basic programs (e.g., accountant/bookkeeping and secretary/administrative assistant) and traditional rural programs (e.g., the building trades, welding, and agriscience) (NCES, 2002). They are less likely to offer programs in health and life science occupations, computers and electronics, or paralegal training, all of which are essential for building not only the health care infrastructure, but also the local economy and community resources. To move forward, rural schools must place greater emphasis on preparing students for the knowledge-based economy by enhancing math and science curricula in both grade school and high school, providing advanced placement classes, expanding vocational training programs, and preparing students for college. Enhanced math and science preparation is critical to preparing rural students to pursue careers in the health professions.

The major gap between rural and urban areas today is in college education (see Table B-2): 15.5 percent of rural adults have a 4-year college degree, compared with 26.6 percent of metro adults. About 41 percent of rural residents have completed 1 or more years of schooling beyond high school, indicating an initial interest in and motivation for higher education.

Demographic and geographic characteristics[10] strongly influence college attainment in rural areas, while the status of the local economy affects whether those with a college degree remain in the community given the smaller proportion of jobs that require advanced education.[11] Rural communities need to fully leverage the availability of local colleges and universities by enhancing their role in bridging the gaps in educational opportuni-

---

[10] Rural non-Hispanic whites are twice as likely to have a college degree as other rural groups, while rural Hispanics have the lowest attainment (about half have not finished high school, and only 1 in 16 has completed 4 years of college). Rural counties located in the South, especially in Appalachia, have the lowest high school completion rates, which coincide with the highest rates of persistent poverty (Ricketts, 2000).

[11] In metropolitan America, 35.2 percent of all employment is in managerial, professional, and related work, versus 26.9 percent in nonmetropolitan areas (including all farm operators/managers).

TABLE B-2　USDA Economic Research Service: Educational Attainment, 2000

Characteristic	Less Than High School		High School Graduate		Some College		College Graduate	
Geographic Status	N[a]	M[b]	N	M	N	M	N	M
African American	31.9	19.0	40.2	34.8	20.2	28.4	7.9	17.9
Hispanic	51.8	42.2	27.3	27.6	15.1	18.5	5.9	11.6
Native American	27.7	18.8	38.9	32.7	25.0	32.6	8.4	16.0
Caucasian[c]	16.7	10.0	40.8	31.7	25.1	26.8	17.4	31.5

[a] N = nonmetropolitan.
[b] M = metropolitan.
[c] Non-Hispanic white population.
SOURCE: Calculated by C. Beale at ERS using data from the 2000 census of the population.

ties for rural students and in lifelong learning for adults. For example, a community college could offer associate degrees in nursing and computer science, and the two departments could develop a partnership to establish an education and support center for local providers implementing health information and communications applications, and for local residents who would like to learn how to use self-care monitoring devices and/or participate in online disease management programs.

Local colleges could also partner with local community libraries to provide residents with a resource for general adult literacy programs, health literacy programs (e.g., locating and understanding health information), and means of overcoming language barriers. A 1993 study by the Rural Clearinghouse for Lifelong Learning and Development found that rural residents account for 42 percent of the functionally illiterate in the United States (based on self-reports on grade level completion).[12] Those at the lowest

---

[12] More substantial national data on literacy statistics, including rural–urban delineations, will be available from the 2003 National Adult Literacy Survey report; publication is expected in 2005.

literacy levels had an eighth-grade education or less, and were more likely to be older (over age 65), disabled, or a member of a minority group (e.g., African American, Native American, Hispanic, Asian or Pacific Islander). Improving local resources to help those with low literacy skills is critical to supporting individuals' ability to understand their health conditions and their role in their treatment plans.

THE DIGITAL DIVIDE

Individuals and communities can no longer grow with the new knowledge-based economy unless they have access to modern high-speed telecommunications networks, computer systems, and the Internet to facilitate their personal and business needs. The knowledge-based economy is changing the way businesses operate and the skills required of the labor force. Likewise, knowledge-based systems are transforming the ways in which individuals can manage their personal needs, including health care.

Nationally, however, a digital divide exists between rural regions and urban communities (Bell et al., 2004). This divide is exacerbated by higher rural infrastructure costs and lower average wages, which generally limit the penetration of new information technologies. Rural areas have less access than urban to digital subscriber line (DSL) and cable modem services, which provide the greater bandwidth needed for many health care applications (see Chapter 6) (Allen, 2001). This aspect of the digital divide is one of the greatest challenges for rural telehealth and other rural commerce.

Internet penetration rates have historically been lower in rural areas (52 percent of the population) than urban (67 percent) or suburban areas (66 percent), but have continued to increase in all geographic areas over time (Bell et al., 2004). The lower penetration rates coincide with the demographic patterns of rural areas—lower-income people, older people, and minorities exhibit lower rates of Internet usage.[13] Internet users in rural areas keep pace with those in other areas: 45 percent of rural Internet users access the Internet daily, versus 40 percent for urban and 46 percent for

---

[13] Senior citizens make up a larger proportion of rural residents but are less likely to go online—only 17 percent of rural seniors use the Internet. Rural African Americans are significantly less likely than rural whites to go online, possibly because of differences in income and education: 54 percent of rural whites go online, versus 31 percent of rural African Americans.

suburban. Compared with their suburban and urban counterparts, rural users are less likely to bank, buy a product, or make a travel reservation online, but they are more likely to look for religious/spiritual information online.

Chapter 6 provides recommendations for increasing rural access to information and telecommunications technology. To encourage their use of the Internet for health purposes, many rural residents will need guidance and assistance in learning how to use computers and disease management databases, search for information appropriate to their level of education, and use other applications. It is imperative that rural communities develop these resources for their populations—perhaps in the form of community telecenters that might be associated with public libraries and local colleges. Understanding and being able to use the Internet for health communications and information retrieval will have a significant impact on access to and the quality of health care services for rural residents, and more important, is necessary for self-care and disease management in the knowledge-based economy.

HEALTH INSURANCE

Against a background of federal and state initiatives to extend health insurance, the proportion of people under 65 without health insurance grew over the period 1987–2002, from 13.7 percent in 1987 to 17.2 percent in 2002 (IOM, 2004). Moreover, despite a favorable economic climate in the 1990s, the uninsured population grew by more than 6 million during the decade. Even at the height of this prosperous period, the number of uninsured dropped by less than a million. In 2000, the uninsured rate began to grow again, and by 2003 there were 43.3 million uninsured people under age 65 (IOM, 2004).

Location is an important factor in rural uninsurance rates. A 2003 report by the Kaiser Commission on Medicaid and the Uninsured notes that (using 1998 data) 24 percent of individuals living in rural, nonadjacent counties are uninsured, compared with 18 percent for urban areas (Ziller et al., 2003). Although they are 50 percent more likely to have Medicaid coverage than residents in urban counties, it is not enough to compensate for the lower private coverage. Two-thirds of the uninsured are low-income families (less than 200 percent of the federal poverty level), and 30 percent are children (Ziller et al., 2003). The result is added pressure on the local health care services in these most rural counties to act as safety net providers. Differences in uninsurance rates between urban counties and those rural counties adjacent to urban counties, as well as between urban and larger nonadjacent counties, were found not to be statistically significant. Health insurance disparities associated with rural residence were found to be related to the structure of employment—specifically smaller employers, lower wages, and greater prevalence of self-employment.

REFERENCES

Allen KC. 2001. *Advanced Telecommunications in Rural America.* [Online]. Available: http://www.its.bldrdoc.gov/tpr/2000/its_t/adv_tele/adv_tele.html [accessed July 7, 2004].

Anderson G, Horvath J. 2002. *Chronic Conditions: Making the Case for Ongoing Care.* Baltimore, MD: Johns Hopkins University and The Robert Wood Johnson Foundation.

Beale C, Cromartie J. 2004 (February). *Profile of the Rural Population.* Commissioned Paper for the IOM Committee on the Future of Rural Health Care. Washington, DC.

Bell P, Reddy P, Raine L. 2004. *Rural Areas and the Internet.* Washington, DC: Pew Internet and American Life Project.

Census (Bureau of the Census). 2003a. *Income in the United States, 2002: Current Population Reports.* Washington, DC: U.S. Bureau of the Census.

Census. 2003b. *2000 Census of Population and Housing: Summary Social, Economic, and Housing Characteristics.* [Online]. Available: http://www.census.gov/census2000/pubs/phc-2.html [accessed June 29, 2004].

CMS (Centers for Medicare and Medicaid Services). 2004. *Fact Sheet: Rural Health Clinics.* [Online]. Available: http://www.cms.hhs.gov/medlearn/rhcfactsheet.pdf [accessed June 30, 2004].

ERS (Economic Research Service). 2002. *Rural America.* Washington, DC: Economic Research Service. P. 16.

ERS. 2003a. *Measuring Rurality: Urban-Rural Continuum Codes.* [Online]. Available: http://www.ers.usda.gov/Briefing/Rurality/RuralUrbCon/ [accessed November 4, 2004].

ERS. 2003b. *Rural Employment and Unemployment.* [Online]. Available: http://www.ers.usda.gov/Briefing/LaborAndEducation/employunemploy/ [accessed March 24, 2004].

ERS. 2003c. *Rural Industry: Which Industries Are Most Important to Rural America?* [Online]. Available: http://ers.usda.gov/Briefing/Industry/importantindust/ [accessed June 29, 2003].

ERS. 2004. *Rural Hispanics: Employment and Residential Trends.* [Online]. Available: http://www.ers.usda.gov/Amberwaves/June04/Features/RuralHispanic.htm [accessed June 25, 2004].

FR (Federal Register). 2000. *Standards for Defining Metropolitan and Micropolitan Statistical Areas.* Washington, DC: Office of Management and Budget.

Gamm L, Hutchison L, Bellamy G, Dabney B. 2002. Rural healthy people 2010: Identifying rural health priorities and models for practice. *Journal of Rural Health* 18(1):9–14.

IOM (Institute of Medicine). 2002. *Care Without Coverage: Too Little Too Late.* Washington, DC: The National Academies Press.

IOM. 2004. *Insuring America's Health: Principles and Recommendations.* Washington, DC: The National Academies Press.

Marshall R. 2004. *Rural Policy in a New Century.* [Online]. Available: http://www.kc.frb.org/PUBLICAT/beyond/RC00Mars.pdf [accessed May 24, 2004].

NCES (National Center for Education Statistics). 2002. *Issue Brief: Vocational Education Offerings in Rural High Schools.* [Online]. Available: http://nces.ed.gov/pubs2002/2002120.pdf [accessed May 24, 2004].

NCHS (National Center for Health Statistics). 2001. *Health, United States, 2001 with Urban and Rural Health Chartbook.* Washington, DC: U.S. Department of Health and Human Services.

OMB (Office of Management and Budget). 2000 (December 27). Standards for Defining Metropolitan and Micropolitan Statistical Areas. [Online]. Available: http://www.census.gov/population/www/estimates/00-32997.pdf

PRB (Population Reference Bureau). 1999. *The Rural Rebound.* [Online]. Available: http://www.prb.org/Content/NavigationMenu/PRB/AboutPRB/Reports_on_America/ReportonAmericaRuralRebound.pdf [accessed May 2004].

Ricketts TC. 1999. *Rural Health in the United States.* New York: Oxford University Press.

Ricketts TC. 2000. The changing nature of rural health care. *Annual Review of Public Health* 21(1):639–657.

Rosenblatt R. 2000. The health of rural people and the communities and environments in which they live. In: Geyman JP, Norris TE, Hart GL, eds. *Textbook of Rural Medicine.* New York: McGraw-Hill. Pp. 3–14.

Zhang W, Bowman A, Mueller K. 1998. *Rural/Urban Definitions: Alternatives and Numbers by State.* Omaha, NE: Nebraska Center for Rural Health Research, University of Nebraska Medical Center.

Ziller E, Coburn A. 2003. *Health Insurance Coverage of the Rural and Urban Near Elderly.* Portland, ME: Maine Rural Health Research Center, University of Southern Maine.

C

The Rural Health Care Delivery System

The quality of the rural health care delivery system is determined by the availability of providers and health care facilities to rural residents and the ability of those providers and organizations to give care that is needed and effective in generating positive health outcomes (Gregg and Moscovice, 2003; Rosenblatt, 2002). The availability of rural providers can vary significantly from one county to another, and many rural communities struggle to provide even basic health care services to their population. Typically, the smaller, poorer, and more isolated the rural community, the more difficult it is to ensure that basic health care needs are met (Rosenblatt, 2002).

In most rural communities, the health care delivery system is a patchwork of primary care providers, clinics, hospitals, and other facilities that function through the private sector either independently in private practice or as part of a network. However, there are fewer health care organizations and professionals of all kinds in rural areas, and less choice and competition among them. Local safety net providers deliver a sizable amount of care to the uninsured, Medicaid enrollees, and other vulnerable populations (IOM, 2000). This appendix provides a brief overview of the rural health care systems for primary care, emergency medical services (EMS), hospital care, long-term care, mental health and substance abuse care, oral health care, and public health.

PRIMARY CARE

Access to primary care is the top-ranking health priority for rural areas (Gamm et al., 2003). Across the health sector, primary care is highly valued as the key mechanism for meeting the majority of health care needs of most individuals. Primary care practices provide essential care for a wide range of health problems; guide patients through the health system, including referrals; foster an ongoing relationship between clinicians and patients (and their families); support disease prevention, management, and health promotion; and build bridges to the local community (IOM, 1996). Shortages in the supply of primary care providers directly affect not only the health status of individuals, but also the rest of the providers in the delivery system.

In rural areas, as in urban, the bulk of health care services are provided in primary care practice settings in the local community, such as small private practices, community health centers, and rural health clinics. The main differences between rural and urban providers are the health professionals engaged in primary care and the scope of practice; the actual structure of urban and rural practice settings tends to be similar.

Primary Care Clinicians

Rural primary care providers are more likely than urban to be family physicians or generalists with a broad scope of practice, and a greater proportion are more likely to be midlevel professionals (e.g., nurse practitioners, physician assistants). The scope of practice for rural physicians can include primary care subspecialties such as pediatrics, obstetrics and gynecology, gerontology, internal medicine, and general surgery for certain procedures, as well as the traditional primary care services for episodic care, preventive care, and chronic disease management. Because certain specialty services are unavailable in rural areas, many rural physicians also provide services characteristic of specialty practice, such as intensive care (51.4 percent), emergency department care (58 percent), and specialist procedures (e.g., sigmoidoscopy [29 percent]) (Phillips and Green, 2002). Some midlevel practitioners provide services in specialist areas as well.

Following is a summary of the presence of these providers in rural practices. As this discussion is limited to clinicians having the greatest contact with patients, pharmacists also are included, but allied health professionals (e.g., laboratory technicians and radiologists) are not. Providers of emergency care, mental health and substance abuse services, and dental care are discussed in their respective sections. A more thorough discussion of the rural health workforce is provided in Chapter 4.

Physicians

Overall, rural areas have a lower complement of physicians than do urban areas. In 2000, there were 119 physicians (including both generalists and specialists) per 100,000 population in rural areas, compared with 225 physicians per 100,000 population in urban areas (Larson et al., 2003). Restricting the analysis to generalist physicians may be a better proxy for physicians providing primary care. Using county-level data, the gap between rural and urban is reduced, with rural areas having about 57 generalist physicians per 100,000 population, compared with 78 generalists per 100,000 population in urban areas. Statewide estimates tend to gloss over the wide variability in provider shortages and surpluses at the individual county level, however. For example, Wisconsin's statewide average of 68 primary physicians per 100,000 population (2000 data) is higher than the national average of 59 per 100,000, but the state's median of county averages is 31 physicians per 100,000 population. This indicates major differences in the distribution of physicians among Wisconsin counties, with many falling far below the statewide and national averages (WHA, 2004). This effect is rather common. A 23 state study confirmed that there were about 35.5 physicians per 100,000 in the most rural areas (Rosenthal et al. 2003). Overall, in 1999, 91 percent of towns with 2,500 to 5,000 population in 23 states had a general practitioner or family physician—a gain of 5 percentage points over 1979 (Rosenthal et al. 2003).

Osteopathic physicians also have a presence in rural areas at 5 percent. Larsen and colleagues (2003) found that osteopaths are more likely to practice as generalists or to become family physicians (46 percent) than are allopathic physicians (11 percent) and more likely to choose to practice in rural areas (18 versus 11.5 percent).

Specialist physicians in rural areas have a relatively low presence compared to their urban counterparts. A study by Baldwin et al. (1999) found that only 6.2 percent of such physicians are located in rural areas. Specifically, 7.9 percent of gastroenterologists, 17.6 percent for general surgeons, 10.8 percent of obstetrics/gynecologists, 12.7 percent of opthalmologists, 12.9 percent of orthopedic surgeons, 13.3 percent of otolaryngologists, and 11 percent of urologists are located in rural areas. Rosenthal et al. (2003) reviewed the growth of specialists in rural communities over a 20-year period, finding sizable growth in the presence of many specialties (see Table C-1). Selected specialties—emergency medicine (19.2 percent) and psychia-

TABLE C-1 Percentage of Communities with Nonfederal Physician Specialty Services 1979–1999

Specialty	Number of Physicians	Population in Thousands		
		2,500–4,999	5,000–9,999	10,000–19,999
General and family practice				
1979	11,869	86	96	99
1999	21,919	91	96	99
Internal medicine				
1979	9,467	23	52	84
1999	20,654	41	69	93
General surgery				
1979	6,071	44	77	96
1999	5,275	38	63	88
Obstetrics and gynecology				
1979	3,978	15	35	77
1999	7,092	15	41	82
Psychiatry				
1979	3,203	9	17	40
1999	6,155	9	26	53
Pediatrics				
1979	3,429	12	25	68
1999	9,356	16	43	84
Radiology				
1979	3,042	9	30	73
1999	4,909	13	36	68
Anesthesiology				
1979	2,303	11	19	40
1999	5,914	7	20	64
Orthopedic surgery				
1979	2,409	7	17	47
1999	3,927	7	28	69
Opthalmology				
1979	2,147	4	14	62
1999	3,328	3	18	60
Pathology				
1979	1,840	4	15	50
1999	2,747	4	13	49
Urology				
1979	1,340	2	10	47
1999	1,879	2	13	57
Otolaryngology				
1979	1,127	2	6	29
1999	1,685	1	10	46
Dermatology				
1979	795	1	3	15
1999	1,475	2	7	33
Neurology				
1979	724	1	4	13
1999	1,901	1	7	28

SOURCE: Rosenthal et al., 2003.

try (4.8 percent)— are discussed in more detail in their respective sections later in this appendix.

Nurse Practitioners

A good deal of primary care also is provided by nurse practioners. Nurse practioner training programs began as certificate-level training for registered nurses, but master's degree training has grown significantly (Berlin et al., 1999). In 2000, there were over 58,000 employed nurse practioners, 22 percent of whom practiced in rural areas (Hooker, 2002). Approximately 85 percent of nurse practioners practice in primary care (Hooker, 2002). Certification requirements established by the American Nurse Credentialing Center ensure that the nurse practioner workforce meets certain standards. However, there is no national dataset comparable to the American Medical Association Physician Masterfile to monitor this workforce in terms of supply, credentials, and where and how they are deployed (Phillips et al., 2002).

Physician Assistants

Physician assistants are health care professionals licensed to practice with physician supervision (AAPA, 2003). In 2000, there were about 45,000 practicing physician assistants, 23 percent practicing in rural areas. Unlike nurse practioners, who for the most part practice in primary care, physician assistants are equally divided between primary and specialty care (usually hospital-based).

For this group of professionals, there is little overall difference in statewide average staffing levels between rural (13 per 100,000 population) and urban counties (14 per 100,000 population) (Larson et al., 2003). Rural areas with relatively low physician assistant staffing ratios are located in the southeastern states (except for West Virginia, with double the average ratio), some of the northeastern states, and a few of the western states.

Pharmacists

In 2000, 196,000 pharmacists were active in the United States (Hart et al., 2002; HRSA, 2000). About 60 percent of pharmacists work in retail or community pharmacies; the remainder work in institutional settings, such as hospitals and clinics. Although increases in the number of pharmacists have outpaced the rate of population growth, rural areas are experiencing supply problems. Comprehensive surveys of urban–rural pharmacist supplies are not available at this time. However, current vacancy rates of up to 18 percent have been noted for the Veterans Administration and the Indian Health Service alone (HRSA, 2000). Other major concerns among many rural pharmacists are the lack of relief coverage and the lack of round-the-clock service availability, particularly in high-demand areas such as those with a large population of elderly residents (Casey et al., 2001).

Primary Care Settings

Most primary care services in rural communities are provided in small private practice settings. According to the American Academy of Family Physicians, physicians practicing independently in groups of four or fewer provide over 70 percent of care throughout the country. Data have not been stratified for rural counties; however, survey data for family and general practice physicians, who constitute about half of physicians in rural areas, indicate that 23 percent practice solo, 10 percent in two-person partnerships, 39 percent in family practice groups of two or more, and 20 percent in multispecialty groups (Personal communication, G. Tolleson, June 2, 2004). More detailed information differentiating rural and urban physician office practices is needed to determine configurations that may be useful as a model for developing the rural health care delivery system.

Some primary care is provided through community health centers and rural health clinics that may qualify through the Centers for Medicare and Medicaid Services for special federal funding programs if they meet certain criteria. In 2002, 428 of the 843 total community health centers were located in rural areas (LaLonde, 1975). Community health centers may qualify under Section 330 of the Public Health Service Act to receive federal grants covering the cost of primary care and support services (e.g., transportation, translation) to low-income people living in medically underserved areas (Bloom et al., 2001). Technical assistance provided through the Health Resources and Services Administration (HRSA) is focused on chronic care management, disease registries, and quality improvement. Sizable expansion of the community health centers program is planned in the next 5 years (BPHC, 2002). While rural health clinics do not receive federal grants, those that maintain a defined set of core services can receive Medicare and Medicaid cost-based reimbursement for care provided by physicians, nurse practitioners, physician assistants, nurse midwives, clinical psychologists, and clinical social workers. As of 2004, about 3,500 rural health clinics were in operation—many of these independent practice providers. Rural health clinics also are a highly valued safety net provider for rural communities, often delivering up to 45 percent of services provided for this purpose (Gale and Coburn, 2003).

EMERGENCY MEDICAL SERVICES

Emergency care encompasses a continuum of health services including prehospital medical services; emergency services provided at the hospital or health center; and the trauma system, which often serves as the network of coordinated care (Probst et al., 1999). Access to and the quality of emergency care, particularly EMS, is a major concern among state offices of rural health and has direct consequences for morbidity and mortality. Efforts to evaluate the quality, status, and utilization of emergency services in specific terms have been hampered by the overall lack of data and the lack of formalized reporting requirements in most states.

Prehospital care is characterized by the availability of ambulance service, quick first-responder rates, and rapid transport times to hospital emergency rooms. Several studies have documented that first-responder rates and transport times are longer in rural areas (Gamm et al., 2003), and rural emergency patients are far more likely to die en route to the hospital than their urban counterparts (Morrisey et al., 1995). Rural EMS confront major challenges including sizable geographic distances between patients and trauma centers and fragmented prehospital transport services, which are usually coordinated more closely with public safety than with the local health care system.

Nationwide data are not available, but some state-specific data and studies indicate that the level of training of emergency medical technicians (EMTs) in rural areas is lower than that in urban areas (Morrisey et al., 1995). There are four primary levels of training for emergency medical technicians:

- First responder—entry-level position for volunteer fire departments, police departments, search-and-rescue teams, and first responder units.
- EMT-basic—entry-level position in EMS ambulance providers that offer basic-level medical and trauma care and limited medications.
- EMT-intermediate—midlevel position in EMS that provides medications and establishes intravenous lines (IVs).
- EMT-paramedic—advanced-level position that provides numerous

medications, IVs, advanced airway procedures, and advanced medical and trauma care.

In many rural communities, EMTs are volunteers, and most are probably trained as first responders. EMT training is generally funded by local tax dollars. Few rural areas can afford a full-time paramedic.

An EMT's skill level is influenced by experience, especially in responding to serious, life-threatening conditions. This is another challenge for rural areas. One study found that rural counties averaged only about 3.3 ambulance runs per week, with 43 percent of runs including the provision of oxygen, one in five establishing an IV line, and only 1.5 percent involving cardiopulmonary resuscitation (Morrisey et al., 1995).

Because of workforce constraints, nearly half of rural hospitals provide emergency care through nurse practitioners and physician assistants. A physician sees the patient concurrently in 50 percent of these emergency departments staffed by midlevel practitioners (one-third to one-fourth of patients) (Williams et al., 2001). It is not uncommon to staff shifts in emergency rooms of small rural hospitals with nurse practioners or physician assistants, with physicians on call for more complex cases. A 1999 survey of 940 short-term acute care hospitals with emergency departments (21 percent rural) found that the average number of physicians available to the emergency department was highest in academic medical centers (13.57) and lowest in rural hospitals (4.74). The vast majority of rural emergency physicians are neither residency trained nor board certified for emergency medicine (39 and 33 percent, respectively, versus 72 percent in both cases in urban hospitals) (Moorhead et al., 2002). In addition, rural physicians' scope of practice entails multitasking and cross-functioning, as they often run outpatient primary care clinics, care for inpatients at their local hospital, serve a role in hospital administration, direct local EMS, and care for patients who present for emergency care (Williams et al., 2001).

Other pressures that compromise the rural emergency care system have been identified and include the lack of or low level of pay for services, lack of universal access to 911 and radio "dead spots" from crowded frequencies, perceptions of increased personal liability, increased exposure to danger (biological, chemical, violence, critical incident stress) in providing EMS, the paucity of rural physicians trained to provide medical supervision of local EMS operations, equipment that tends to be old and dated, lack of leadership, and scarcity of resources to support EMS systems (OMB, 2000). These factors pose severe challenges for the provision of quality emergency

TABLE C-2 Federal Allocations to States for Domestic Preparedness

Name of program	Fiscal Year 2002 State Domestic Preparedness Program	Fiscal Year 2003 State Homeland Security Grant Program I	Fiscal Year 2003 State Homeland Security Grant Program II
Total allocation	$315.7 million	$566.3 million	$1.3 million
Total EMS allocation	$11 million	$21.1 million	$18.3 million
Average EMS allocation	$250,526	$458,886	$542,649
Median EMS allocation	$114,694	$226,467	$333,495

SOURCE: ODP, 2004.

care, from first response through initial stabilization and subsequent treatment (OTA, 1989; Rawlinson and Crews, 2003).

The lack of a national coordinated strategy or infrastructure for EMS has left most systems unprepared and fragmented. The majority of EMS systems are regulated by state health departments (71 percent) or other agencies (e.g., governor's office, public safety department, EMS advisory council) (24 percent) according to figures from July 1989, yet fewer than 31 percent of states have a coordinated statewide EMS plan, and most operate in silos from the local level. The lack of funding has a significant impact on the current state of rural EMS systems. After initial sizable investments by the federal government beginning in 1966, funding for such systems essentially ended in 1981 (USDOT, 1998). Currently, new federal grant programs for domestic preparedness are supplying increased resources to states to enhance emergency responder capabilities (including EMS) and critical infrastructure that will assist local communities in addressing many of these problems (Mohr, 2003). All 50 states and territories have received three allocations, as outlined in Table C-2; however, states need to accelerate the allocation of funds to the local community. In addition, training for first responders is being provided through the National Domestic Preparedness Consortium, as well as other training partners.

Areas of immediate improvement are also part of federal initiatives such as HRSA's program to allocate up to $25 million in grants to rural areas for the purchase, placement, and training in the use of automated external defibrillators in rural communities (HRSA, 2003). Lasting improvement in the quality of EMS will require that new programs be designed with evidence-based standards and procedures, a systems approach to functions and operations, implementation of cutting-edge information and communications technology and telemedicine systems to supplement care, and clearly defined methods for measuring quality and outcomes. An IOM study on EMS and emergency room care is currently in progress, with a series of reports to be released in 2005–2006.

HOSPITAL CARE

In the majority of rural communities, the hospital is the central focus of health care delivery, often providing outpatient, home health, skilled nursing, and other long-term care in addition to inpatient care. Hospitals have had a major role in ensuring the provision of health services in rural areas where no other providers are available, and have been an essential part of the social and economic identity of the local community, often constituting the largest or second-largest employer in the area (Moscovice and Stensland, 2002). Statistics from the American Hospital Association's (AHA) 2000 Annual Survey indicate that, of the total of 4,927 nonfederal, acute care community hospitals in the United States, 44 percent or 2,178 are located in rural counties. Over 70 percent of hospitals with 100 or fewer beds are located in rural areas (see Table C-3) (Colgan, 2002).

TABLE C-3   Hospitals in Rural Areas, Year 2000

Hospitals by Bed Size	Rural	Urban
Under 25	255	66
25–49	711	220
50–99	655	417

SOURCE: Colgan, 2002.

The structure, function, and role of hospitals in the U.S. health care system have been changing rapidly and significantly. From the 1980s through the mid-1990s, about 1,072 hospitals were confronting serious financial difficulties and were forced to close, convert, or merge; of these, 438 were rural (Ricketts, 1999). Rather than close down, many rural hospitals converted to modified inpatient health care facilities and expanded outpatient services (Ricketts, 1999).

Congress responded by establishing the Medicare Rural Hospital Flexibility Program in 1997 (MedPAC, 2004). The "Flex Program" supports critical access hospitals (CAHs) which are limited-service hospitals located in rural areas having up to 25 beds and providing 24-hour emergency care and short-stay (up to 96 hours) inpatient services (CMS, 2004). With the Flex Program, the number of CAHs has grown substantially—to 928 as of May 2004. Fully 90 percent of CAHs are located in medically underserved areas, where there are fewer residents per square mile and a higher proportion of those over age 65 (see Figure C-1) (Doeksen et al., 1997; FMT, 2004a; HRSA, 2004). More specifically, 42 percent are located in areas of <2,500 population, 28 percent in frontier areas. Although the average volume is relatively low at 4.6 patients per day, hospitals that converted in 1999 have been able to maintain modest profit margins. For example, at conversion, average total margins were negative 2.5 percent, then rose to positive 2.3 percent 1 year after conversion and to positive 3.7 percent 2 years after (Stensland et al., 2004). To expand their revenue base further, many CAHs are building networks with other provider groups and adding outpatient services (e.g., mammography, pharmacy, radiology, pathology, surgery, rehabilitation).

Rural hospitals struggle, even more so than urban, to attract and maintain adequate numbers of nurse professionals. Rural counties lag behind urban in the number of full-time, hospital-based registered nurses, with rural counties having 213 registered nurses per 100,000 population as compared with 281 per 100,000 for urban counties (see Figure C-2). Rural hospitals also are more dependent upon various types of advance practice nurses, such as nurse anesthetists, who provide anesthesia services in about two-thirds of rural hospitals (AANA, 2004). Workforce supply is a key issue for many rural hospitals, discussed extensively in Chapter 4.

LONG-TERM CARE

Long-term care encompasses a diverse array of services provided over a sustained period of time to people of all ages with chronic conditions (IOM, 2001). Long-term care ranges from minimal personal assistance with basic, everyday activities to skilled nursing care, and can be provided in a variety of settings, including nursing homes, residential care facilities, and people's homes.

Most users of long-term care facilities are individuals over age 65 (IOM, 2001). A 2000 study found that over 9 million individuals aged 65+ resided in rural counties; 4.3 million of these were aged 75+ and most likely to use

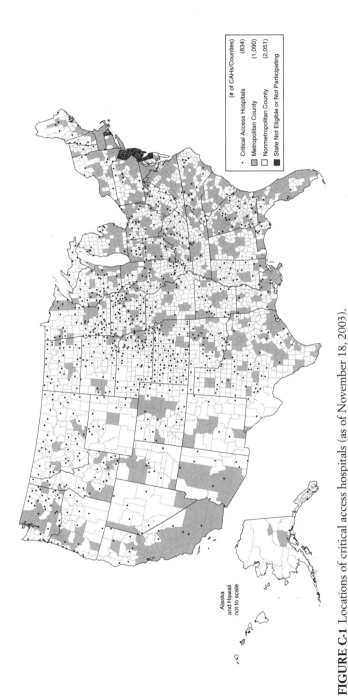

FIGURE C-1 Locations of critical access hospitals (as of November 18, 2003).

NOTE: Developed with data from the U.S. Census Bureau (2003); U.S. Department of Health and Human Services, Centers for Medicare and Medicaid (CMS) (2003); and CMS Regional Office, Office of Rural Health Policy, and State Officers Coordinating with Medicare Rural Health Flex Program (2004). Core Based Statistical Areas (CBSA) are current as of the December 2003 update. Nonmetropolitan counties include micropolitan and counties outside of CBSAs. Produced by: North Carolina Rural Health Research and Policy Analysis Center, Cecil G. Sheps Center for Health Services Research, University of North Carolina at Chapel Hill.

SOURCE: FMT, 2004b.

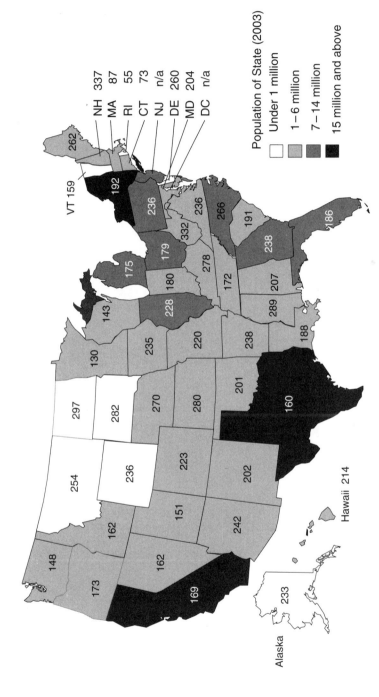

FIGURE C-2 Full-time, hospital-based registered nurses per 100,000 population (average for each state's rural counties, 2,000).
SOURCE: Larson and Norris, 2003.

nursing homes in the near future (Phillips et al., 2003). Rural elders differ from their urban counterparts in several ways: they are more likely to be poor and less educated, to live in homes that are substandard (although fully owned), to lack health insurance coverage, and to be in poor health (Coward et al., 1994; Ricketts, 1999).

Long-term care in rural areas is characterized by greater reliance on institutionally based care in hospitals and nursing homes than is the case in urban areas. About one of every four U.S. residents aged 75 or older lives in rural America, yet over 40 percent of the nation's nursing home beds are in rural areas (NRHA, 2001a; Phillips et al., 2003). Utilization of nursing homes is highest in small towns (121.5 nursing home residents for every 1,000 persons aged 75 and older) and lowest in urban areas (82.3 nursing home residents), but even isolated areas (99.0 nursing home residents) and large towns (106.7 nursing home residents) see higher use of nursing homes among the very old than that in urban areas (Phillips et al., 2003). If alternatives to institutional care, such as assisted living facilities, were available, about $2–$5 billion in Medicaid spending could be saved per year (Clark, 1998).

Although older rural residents are more likely to use nursing home care, such care in rural areas differs from that in urban areas in two ways. First, nursing homes located in rural areas are less likely to have certified skilled nursing beds or special care units; they provide mainly custodial care (Ricketts, 1999). Second, nursing homes in rural areas have lower staffing ratios for both nurse aides and licensed nursing staff (Abt Associates, 2001). Physical therapists and social workers are also in short supply given the higher incidence of disability and frailty among rural residents (Ricketts, 1999).

Quality concerns have been raised regarding the care provided in both urban and rural nursing homes and the adequacy of oversight mechanisms (MedPAC, 2001), but these concerns may be even greater for rural facilities. A large proportion of rural nursing homes have nurse staffing ratios that fall below the minimum considered essential for the delivery of safe care (Phillips et al., 2003). (See Chapter 4 for further discussion of the challenges rural areas confront in recruiting an adequate nursing workforce.) Rural nursing home patients are also more likely to experience multiple transfers from nursing facility to hospital, an indication that rural facilities experience difficulty in managing medically complex patients (Coburn et al., 1999). Data and information are less plentiful on differences in the availability, use, or quality of home health care in rural versus urban areas. According to recent Medicare claims data (which pertain to post–acute care, short-term home health use), urban and rural providers treat a clinically similar mix of patients—Alzheimer's disease, congestive heart failure, diabetes, stroke, hip procedure and fracture, and chronic obstructive pulmonary disease—with similar functional status (MedPAC, 2001). Rural patients received more total visits (43.8 per year) than their urban counterparts (37.5 per year), but fewer rural patients received therapy visits. Studies of the quality of home health care generally do not differentiate between rural and urban areas, but there is a sizable evidence base documenting safety and quality shortcomings in home health care overall (GAO, 1997; IOM, 2001).

MENTAL HEALTH AND SUBSTANCE ABUSE CARE

After access to primary care, access to mental health services is cited by Gamm and colleagues (2003) as the second-highest priority for improving rural health delivery system. In both urban and rural areas, a growing portion of mental health services are being provided by primary care clinicians, but for different reasons. Mental health conditions[1] cover a wide range of conditions and severity—from those that are less severe, such as generalized anxiety disorder, to those that are more severe, such as schizophrenia. Substance abuse[2] refers to dependence upon and excessive consumption of alcohol, illicit drugs, and/or tobacco. Although mental health conditions and substance abuse have traditionally been associated with different treatment settings, program and funding mechanisms, and research literatures, there is increasing evidence that many individuals have both conditions as each is an

---

[1] For the purposes of this discussion, mental illness, mental disorders, and serious mental illness are distinguished as follows: *mental illness* refers to all diagnosable mental disorders (USDHHS, 2000); *mental disorders* include schizophrenia, affective disorders such as depression, and anxiety disorders such as bipolar disorder (Regier et al., 1993); *serious mental illness* is a diagnosable mental disorder found in persons aged 18 and older that is so long-lasting and severe that it seriously interferes with a person's ability to take part in major life activities (USDHHS, 2000); *serious emotional disturbance* is a diagnosable mental disorder found in persons from birth to age 18 that is so severe and long-lasting that it seriously interferes with functioning in family, school, community, or other major life activities (USDHHS, 2000).

[2] Substance abuse includes alcohol, tobacco, and illicit drug use. Although alcohol and tobacco are by far the two most prevalently abused substances and are significant causes of morbidity and mortality (Hutchison and Blakely, 2003), abuse of alcohol and illicit drugs frequently co-occurs with mental illness (Barry et al., 1996; Coridan and Heffron 2000 [Updated Spring 2002]). Marijuana is the most commonly used illicit drug, followed by cocaine and hallucinogens.

important contributor to the other and to other serious medical conditions, and effective treatment of either requires attention to the other by providers that have competency in the behavioral and social treatment of both.

Mental health conditions and substance abuse exact high social costs (potentially long-term) and financial costs that other illnesses typically do not impose for families, communities, and legal systems, as they are the leading causes of disability-related conditions.[3] Access to care and support mechanisms for patients and their families are critically important to appropriate treatment and management of these conditions; however, adequate services are often not available. Primary care providers often fill the gap in mental health services in rural areas. In contrast, cost and limited coverage of mental health and substance abuse services deter many urban patients from seeking out primary care providers for these services.

Recent estimates indicate that about 16.5 percent of the U.S. population over age 18 have a mental disorder and 7.6 percent a substance abuse disorder in any given year (Narrow et al., 2002). The 1999 Surgeon General's report estimated that 20 percent of children had mental disorders with mild functional impairment, with a subset of 5–9 percent having severe functional limitations (USPHS, 1999). The prevalence of mental health conditions and substance abuse in rural areas is comparable to that in urban areas, with some notable exceptions (Hartley et al., 1999; Kessler et al., 1994; NCHS, 2001). Rural areas suffer from a higher incidence of suicide and suicide attempts than their urban counterparts; rural residents are less likely to request care for mental health (Fox et al., 1999; Rost et al., 2002); and rural youth have higher rates of abuse of alcohol, tobacco, methamphetamines, and inhalants (Butterfield et al., 2002; Donnermeyer and Scheer, 2001; Hutchison and Blakely, 2003; OAS, 2003).

The rural elderly, who constitute a larger portion of the rural than the urban population, have a higher incidence of depression compared with other populations—particularly those with multiple chronic conditions taking four or more medications (Crystal et al., 2003; Okwumabua et al., 1997). Rural women are at greater risk for depression and stress-related disorders than rural men, and these conditions are less likely to be diagnosed by a rural practitioner (Shelton et al., 1995). The rate of substance abuse is lower for women than for men in general; however, rural women experience greater severity of alcohol problems, more comorbidities, and more deleterious con-

---

[3] Mental illnesses and substance abuse rank first and second as leading causes of disability-related conditions.

sequences of substance abuse relative to urban women. Children with mental health conditions, substance abuse, or dual diagnosis are 2–4 times more likely to be children of poverty, the welfare system, or the juvenile system (Glied et al., 1997). Some minorities who reside in rural areas, such as Native Americans and Alaska Natives, have a higher incidence of abuse for certain substances (Freese et al., 2000). For example, the alcohol-related death rate among Alaska Natives is 34 per 100,000, compared with 14 per 100,000 for the U.S. population overall (Stillner et al., 1999). The association of mental health conditions and substance abuse with stigma is stronger in rural areas, where there is less anonymity and more overlap in social settings (religious, professional, and personal) (NFCMH, 2003). As a result, rural residents are less likely to have knowledge about mental health conditions and substance abuse, perceive the need for care, and participate in care (Fortney and Booth, 2001).

Access to mental health and substance abuse services varies widely by population density, with rural residents facing a distinct disparity in scope and availability of services (Donnermeyer, 1997). While urban populations can navigate through a variety of treatments offered by multiple providers to gain the necessary care, rural populations must rely on the limited medical and behavioral therapeutic support available to them. Mental health and substance abuse professionals can include psychiatrists (specialist physicians), clinical psychologists, counselors, social workers, and therapists with master's level training (Ivey et al., 1998). All of these providers, particularly those with master's level training, are in short supply in rural areas. Data show that 87 percent of the 1,669 mental health professions shortage areas are rural counties. Of the 1,253 rural counties with populations of 2,500–20,000, 75 percent have no psychiatrist, and only 50 percent have a clinical psychologist or social worker (Bird et al., 2001).[4] This averages to fewer than 2 specialty mental health organizations per rural

---

[4] A federally designated mental health professions shortage area includes rural communities (a catchment area as defined by state mental health planners) with less than 1 psychiatrist per 30,000 population, 1 mental health provider (physician, clinical psychologist, clinical social worker, advanced practice psychiatric nurse, or marriage and family therapist) per 9,000 persons, or a combination of less than 1 psychiatrist per 20,000 population and 1 mental health provider per 6,000 persons. These ratios are lower for areas with greater than average needs (poverty, relatively greater numbers of youth or elders, prevalence of alcohol or substance abuse). Designation as a shortage area qualifies a rural community to receive a National Health Service Corps or state placement, as well as making it eligible for other workforce programs.

county, compared with 13+ such organizations in urban areas (Hartley et al., 1999). A full 20 percent of rural counties lack any mental health services, versus 5 percent of urban. Rural children with serious mental illness are particularly disadvantaged in obtaining the care they need, given a lack of specialized mental health professionals for children and adolescents (Wolff et al., 2001). Moreover, fewer rural than urban hospitals offer inpatient psychiatric services[5] (Hartley et al., 1999). Consequently, primary care clinicians provide mental health services annually for 10 to 20 percent of those living in rural areas (DeGruy, 1996; Ivey et al., 1998) and up to 65 percent of those living in frontier areas (Mohatt et al., 2003). On average nationally, 6 percent of generalists provide mental health services (USPHS, 1999).

The types of organizations that provide care are rather sparse as well. Community mental health centers were created by Congress in 1963 to provide a broad range of mental health services to people regardless of their ability to pay. These facilities have been an important source of mental health and substance abuse services for many rural communities, but less so in recent years. Although community mental health centers were quite effective in reintegrating patients discharged from institutional mental health settings back into the community, a shift to block grants, funding cuts, and the movement toward deinstitutionalization caused many of these facilities to shift their focus to care solely for severely impaired adults and children (Wagenfeld et al., 1994). Because the federal government no longer provides direct support to these centers, official federal designation as a community mental health center is no longer provided, and all qualification requirements to receive financial support are determined by the state.

Treatment for substance abuse is funded largely by the public sector, with 90 percent of such care provided through a diverse range of outpatient settings (e.g., hospitals—10 percent, residential facilities—19 percent, community mental health centers—18.7 percent, and other outpatient settings—44.2 percent)[6] (Horgan and Levine, 1998). Only 2 percent of substance

---

[5] Although the effectiveness of inpatient hospital mental health care for children is increasingly questioned (Glied and Cuellar, 2003) and some state mental hospitals may be underutilized, there are widely published accounts of a lack of needed psychiatric beds as the existing supply is reduced in response to declining reimbursement levels (Appelbaum, 2003).

[6] Nationally, about one-quarter of metropolitan hospitals provide outpatient treatment for alcohol and drug abuse; in rural areas, however, only one-tenth offer such services (CASA [National Center on Addiction and Substance Abuse], 2000).

abuse treatment centers are located in rural areas and most often within a community health center, compared with 9 to 21 percent for urban areas (SAMHSA, 2003). More recently, the Bureau of Primary Health Care has been expanding the role of federally qualified community health centers in mental health and substance abuse services[7] for underserved populations, in recognition of the fact that between 1996 and 2001, mental health and substance abuse encounters in community health centers grew by over 50 percent[8] (Lambert and Agger, 1995; Williams, 2003).

Rural programs that aim to increase workforce capacity have been most successful by adjusting the regulatory and financing framework to better support the training, recruitment, and retention of master's-level practitioners. As discussed in Chapter 4, developing a workforce of advanced practice psychiatric nurses, is one method for increasing the supply of mental health clinicians in rural areas (Hartley et al., 2004; Merwin and Mauck, 1995). Another method is to offer additional training and reimbursement to primary care clinicians who provide mental health services to better support them in this role. Improved data collection on all clinicians providing mental health and substance abuse services also is important and would generate an understanding of the distribution and quality of these services in meeting the needs of rural patients. The IOM's forthcoming study on access to and quality of mental health and substance abuse services will be available in fall 2005.

ORAL HEALTH CARE

In 2000, the Surgeon General published the report Oral Health in America, reestablishing that oral health is essential to the general health and well-being of all individuals and that the two are inseparable. Oral health includes not only the teeth, gums, and surrounding tissues, but also the hard and soft palate; the musocal lining of the mouth, throat, tongue, and lips; the

---

[7] Federally qualified health centers' primary health services are viewed as appropriate for preventing, screening, diagnosing, treating, and managing all forms of common mental illness, such as depression, anxiety, and attention deficit hyperactivity disorder (ADHD). However, their role is viewed as limited to treatment and follow-up for more severe mental disorders, such as schizophrenia, bipolar disorder, or psychotic depression, once these illnesses have been diagnosed and stabilized by specialists (BPHC, 2003).

[8] Some Medicaid Managed Behavioral Healthcare arrangements have been creative in sharing scare mental health professionals by including community mental health centers in networks of providers as well as supporting primary care providers in supplying mental health services.

salivary glands; the chewing muscles; and the upper and lower jaws. Equally important are the nervous, immune, and vascular systems that animate, protect, and nourish the oral tissues, and provide connections to the brain and the rest of the body (USPHS, 2000). The Surgeon General's report confirms that oral health means much more than healthy teeth—it means being free of chronic oral–facial pain conditions, oral and throat cancers, oral soft tissue lesions, birth defects (e.g., cleft lip and palate), and scores of other diseases and disorders that affect the oral, dental, and craniofacial tissues. Oral exams play a critical role in the detection of nutritional deficiencies, as well as a number of systemic diseases (e.g., microbial infections, immune disorders, injuries, and some cancers). Oral health is often overlooked as an important contributor to overall health and in times of high health care costs, is often abdicated to pay for general health care services. Inadequate access to oral health care results in significant financial costs and expenses that go beyond dental diseases.

Despite significant gains over the past 50 years in understanding of the common oral diseases and in dental care, lack of access to oral health care has led to a "silent epidemic" for many vulnerable populations, particularly poor children, the elderly, and many members of racial and ethnic groups (USPHS, 2000). Socioeconomic status and ability to pay are the most influential factors in determining access to oral health care services. The prevalence of dental caries (cavities) is twice as high among low-income than other children, and only 3 percent of rural children receive dental sealants, versus 23 percent of children overall. Racial disparities also are evident among children: 36 percent of African American and 43 percent of Hispanic children have untreated dental caries, compared with 26 percent of whites (ODPHP, 2000). Periodontal disease is more frequent in African Americans and low-income adults—35 percent of adults with less than high school education versus 28 percent of high school graduates and 15 percent of those with some college (Cho, 2000). Rural low-income seniors record higher rates of total tooth loss (47 percent) compared with seniors near metropolitan areas (34 percent) (NCHS, 2001). Data also indicate that 11 percent of rural residents have never seen a dentist (NRHA, 2001b). According to the Rural Healthy People 2010 report, oral health ranked fifth among 28 health areas as a priority for improvement in access and quality for 35 percent of respondents, especially state organizations, community health centers and rural health centers, public health agencies, and hospitals (Gamm et al., 2002).

As with issues related to other health care providers, rural areas are marked by a lack of access to dental services resulting from an inadequate supply of dentists, including those who accept Medicaid or other discounted fee schedules; reluctance of dentists to participate in managed care programs; and the absence of a coordinated screening and referral network (NRHA, 2001b). In metropolitan areas, there are about 43 dentists per 100,000 population, compared with 29 in rural counties, or about 1 dentist per 3,448 residents[9] (Larson et al., 2003). A survey of dental practices in the rural areas of four states (Alabama, California, Maine, and Missouri) found a relatively stable, aging workforce (average ages of 50 years or greater) whose members had practiced in the same location for an average of 16 years (California) to 20 years (Missouri), usually with assistance from both dental hygienists and chair-side dental assistants (Larson and Norris, 2003). Over 60 percent of respondents in all four states identified significant unmet need for dental care in their communities.

Access to oral health care is also impeded by financial barriers. Public health insurance programs (i.e., Medicare, Medicaid, the State Children's Health Insurance Program) do not cover routine dental care, and Medicare provides coverage only for services received in conjunction with inpatient care (CMS, 2001). With the increased funding received in recent years, some community health centers have expanded their services to include dental care. For example, the Midtown community health center in Weber County, Utah, received federal funding for dental care in 2002 and created a partnership with the local university's (Weber State University) dental hygiene program (Nichols, 2004). The university offered the community two offices for dental care at minimal cost, and in exchange the Midtown dentist provides supervision for the dental hygiene students, who provide preventive care and patient education for free as part of their curriculum. Another example involves the community health center of Central Wyoming, which obtained funding through a grant from HRSA and the City of Casper to establish a center for oral health care (North, 2004). This community health center sponsors a dental residency program with dental schools in neighboring states.

---

[9] The federal government designates a health professions shortage area for dentistry if a rural area (county, part of a county, or group of counties with populations at least 40 minutes' travel time apart) has fewer than 1 dentist per 5,000 persons, or fewer than 1 dentist per 4,000 population for areas with greater than average need (at least 20 percent of the population earning less than the federal poverty line, lack of a fluoridated water supply) or insufficient provider capacity (in terms of the number of appointments per dentist annually, the availability of appointments, and average waiting times) (BHPR, 2004).

BOX C-1
Ten Essential Public Health Services

1. Monitor health status to identify community health problems.
2. Diagnose and investigate health problems and health hazards in the community.
3. Inform, educate, and empower people about health issues.
4. Mobilize community partnerships to identify and solve health problems.
5. Develop policies and plans that support individual and community health efforts.
6. Enforce laws and regulations that protect health and ensure safety.
7. Link people to needed personal health services, and ensure the provision of health care when otherwise unavailable.
8. Ensure a competent public health and personal health workforce.
9. Evaluate the effectiveness, accessibility, and quality of personal and population-based health services.
10. Conduct research to obtain new insights and develop innovative solutions to health problems.

SOURCE: NACRHHS, 2000.

PUBLIC HEALTH

Public health services are provided through the state-level agency and by local public health agencies (LPHAs) at the county level, as well as some hospitals, private practice physicians, and community groups. The characteristics of the local community determine which organizations provide these services. In general, a paucity of data has been collected on a regular basis regarding the rural public health infrastructure; the data that are available focus on LPHAs. State public health agencies have been responsible primarily for overall immunization programs, infectious disease control and reporting, health education, health statistics, and most important the licensing and regulation of institutional and individual providers that deliver health care services. However, most services are provided by LPHAs that serve a single county, or in certain cases multiple counties (i.e., large geographic areas in the western United States). About 3,000 LPHAs form the public health system; two-thirds of these are located in small towns with populations of less than 50,000 and median annual expenditures of $621,000 (ORHP, 2002). Some states (e.g., Maine, Pennsylvania) have no LPHAs outside of major cities, and in those that do, the agencies lack personnel and financial resources for population health interventions and enhanced surveillance capabilities. Moreover, workforce recruitment and retention are more difficult in rural areas because of the geographic distance, fewer educational and training opportunities, and less technology diffusion. Efforts are under way by the U.S. Department of Health and Human Services (DHHS) to develop the rural public health infrastructure.

In 1994, the Public Health Functions Working Group, an expert committee convened by DHHS, identified 10 essential public health services (see Box C-1). Earlier IOM committees have recommended that these essential services be available to all communities, regardless of how small or remote they may be (IOM, 1988, 1992, 1997a, 1997b; NRC, 2002). Yet the public health system remains underfunded, and the country lacks a comprehensive, long-term plan to build and sustain this infrastructure at the state and local levels (IOM, 2003). Rural areas often have little or no public health infrastructure (Johnson and Morris, 2000).

REFERENCES

AANA (American Association of Nurse Anesthetists). 2004. *Nurse Anesthetists at a Glance.* [Online]. Available: http://www.aana.com/crna/ataglance.asp [accessed June 30, 2004].

AAPA (American Academy of Physician Assistants). 2003. *2003 AAPA Physician Assistant Census Report.* [Online]. Available: http://www.aapa.org/research/03census-intro.html [accessed April 6, 2004].

Abt Associates. 2001. *Appropriateness of Minimum Nurse Staffing Ratios in Nursing Homes, Phase II Final Report.* [Online]. Available: http://nccnhr.newc.com/uploads/ExecutiveSummary.pdf [accessed June 30, 2004].

Appelbaum PS. 2003. The "quiet" crisis in mental health services. *Health Affairs* 22(5):110–116.

Baldwin LM, Rosenblatt RA, Schneeweiss R, Lishner DM, Hart G. 1999. Rural and urban physicians: Does the content of their Medicare practices differ? *Journal of Rural Health* 15(2):240–251.

Barry KL, Fleming MF, Greenley JR, Kropp S, Widlak P. 1996. Characteristics of persons with severe mental illness and substance abuse in rural areas. *Psychiatric Services* 47(1):88–90.

Berlin LE, Bednash G, Scott D. 1999. *1998–1999 Enrollment and Graduations in Baccalaureate and Graduate Programs in Nursing.* Washington, DC: American Association of Colleges of Nursing.

BHPR (Bureau of Health Professions). 2004. *Health Professional Shortage Area Dental Designation Criteria.* [Online]. Available: http://bhpr.hrsa.gov/shortage/hpsacritdental.htm [accessed April 21, 2004].

Bird DC, Dempsey, P, Hartley, D. 2001. *Addressing Mental Health Workforce Needs in Underserved Rural Areas: Accomplishments and Challenges.* Portland, ME: Maine Rural Health Research Center, University of Southern Maine.

Bloom D, Canning D, Sevilla, J. 2001 (November). *The Effect of Health on Economic Growth: Theory and Evidence.* New York: National Bureau of Economic Research.

BPHC (Bureau of Primary Health Care). 2002. *President's Initiative to Expand Health Centers.* [Online]. Available: http://bphc.hrsa.gov/pinspals/pals.htm [accessed June 2, 2004].

BPHC. 2003. *Opportunities for Health Centers to Expand/Improve Access to Mental Health and Substance Abuse, Oral Health, Pharmacy Services, and Quality Care Management Services During Fiscal Year 2003.* [Online]. Available: ftp://ftp.hrsa.gov/bphc/docs/2003pins/2003-03.pdf [accessed January 8, 2004].

Butterfield P, Malliarakis K, Dotson JA. 2002. Billings' methamphetamine epidemic: Nursing leaders frame a public health and environmental health problem. *Nursing Leadership Forum* 7(1):8–11.

CASA (National Center on Addiction and Substance Abuse). 2000. *CASA Whitepaper: No Place to Hide: Substance Abuse in Mid-Size Cities and Rural America.* Washington, DC: U.S. Conference of Mayors. Notes: Funded by DEA and NIDA.

Casey M, Klingner J, Moscovice I. 2001 (July). *Access to Rural Pharmacy Services in Minnesota, North Dakota, and South Dakota.* Minneapolis, MN: Rural Health Research Center, University of Minnesota.

Cho I. 2000. Disparity in our nation's health: Improving access to oral health care for children. *New York State Dental Journal* 66(9):34–37.

Clark R. 1998. *A New Living Choice for the Elderly.* [Online]. Available: http://www.agenet.com [accessed June 1, 2004].

CMS (Centers for Medicare and Medicaid Services). 2001. *FAQs about Medicare Coverage: Does Medicare Cover Dental Services.* [Online]. Available: http://medicare.custhelp.com/cgi-bin/medicare.cfg/php/enduser/std_adp.php?p_sid=jrzwNdfh&p_lva=&p_faqid=56&p_created=994055331&p_sp=cF9zcm NoPTEm cF9ncmlkc29ydD0mcF9yb3dfY250PTcxJnBfc2VhcmNoX3RleHQ9JnBfc2Vhcm NoX3R5cGU9MyZwX2NhdF9sdmwxPTEyJnBfY2F0X2x2bDI9fmFueX4mc F9zb3J0J0X2J5PWRmbHQmcF9wYWdl PTE*&p_li= [accessed June 30, 2004].

CMS. 2004. *Fact Sheet: Critical Access Hospitals.* [Online]. Available: http://www.cms.hhs.gov/medlearn/cahfactsheet.pdf [accessed July 26, 2004].

Coburn A, Keith R, Bolda E. 1999. *Multiple Hospitalizations Among Elderly Nursing Facility Residents: Is Rural Residence a Risk Factor?* Portland, ME: Maine Rural Health Research Center, University of Southern Maine.

Colgan CS. 2002. *The Economic Effects of Rural Hospital Closures.* Portland, ME: Maine Rural Health Research Center, University of Southern Maine.

Coridan C, Heffron J. 2000 (Updated Spring 2002). *Substance Abuse Parity: A Guide for Advocates.* [Online]. Available: www.nmha.org/state/parity/SAParity.pdf [accessed December 7, 2004].

Coward R, McLaughlin D, Duncan RP. 1994. *An Overview of Health and Aging in Rural America.* Coward R, Brill GK, eds. New York: Springer. Ch. 1.

Crystal S, Sambamoorthi U, Walkup JT, Akincigil A. 2003. Diagnosis and treatment of depression in the elderly Medicare population: Predictors, disparities, and trends. *Journal of the American Geriatric Society* 51(12):1718–1728.

DeGruy F. 1996. *Mental Health Care in the Primary Care Setting.* Washington, DC: National Academy Press.

Doeksen G, Johnson T, Willoughby C. 1997 (January). *Measuring the Economic Importance of the Health Sector on a Local Economy: A Brief Literature Review and Procedures to Measure Local Impacts.* Stillwater, OK: Oklahoma Cooperative Extension, Oklahoma State University.

Donnermeyer JF. 1997. The economic and social costs of drug abuse among the rural population. *NIDA Research Monograph* 168:220–245.

Donnermeyer JF, Scheer SD. 2001. An analysis of substance use among adolescents from smaller places. *Journal of Rural Health* 17(2):105–113.

FMT (Flex Monitoring Team). 2004a. *CAH Information: Complete List of Critical Access Hospitals.* [Online]. Available: http://flexmonitoring.org/cahlist [accessed July 7, 2004].

FMT. 2004b. Location of Critical Access Hospitals. [Online]. Available: http://www.flexmonitoring.org/documents/CAH061004.pdf [accessed July 15, 2004].

Fortney JC, Booth BM. 2001. Access to substance abuse services in rural areas. *Recent Developments in Alcoholism* 15:177–197.

Fox JC, Berman J, Blank M, Rovnyak VG. 1999. Mental disorders and help seeking in a rural impoverished population. *International Journal of Psychiatry in Medicine* 29(2):181–195.

Freese TE, Obert J, Dickow A, Cohen J, Lord RH. 2000. Methamphethamine abuse: Issues for special populations. *Journal of Psychoactive Drugs* 32(2):177–182.

Gale JA, Coburn AF. 2003. *The Characteristics and Roles of Rural Health Clinics in the United States: A Chartbook.* Portland, ME: Maine Rural Health Research Center, University of Southern Maine.

Gamm L, Hutchison L, Bellamy G, Dabney B. 2002. Rural healthy people 2010: Identifying rural health priorities and models for practice. *Journal of Rural Health* 18(1):9–14.

Gamm L, Hutchison L, Dabney B, Dorsey A. 2003. *Rural Healthy People 2010: A Companion Document to Healthy People 2010. Volume 1.* College Station, TX: Texas A&M University System Health Science Center, School of Rural Public Health, Southwest Rural Health Research Center.

GAO (General Accounting Office). 1997 (December). *Medicare Home Health Agencies: Certification Process Ineffective in Excluding Problem Agencies.* [Online]. Available: http://www.gao.gov/archive/1998/he98029.pdf [accessed July 12, 2004].

Glied S, Cuellar AE. 2003. Trends and issues in child and adolescent mental health. *Health Affairs* 22(5):39–50.

Glied S, Hoven CW, Moore RE, Garrett AB, Regier DA. 1997. Children's access to mental health care: Does insurance matter? *Health Affairs* 16(1):67–174.

Gregg W, Moscovice I. 2003. The evolution of rural health networks: Implications for health care managers. *Health Care Management Review* 28(2):161–177.

Hart LG, Salsberg E, Phillips DM, Lishner DM. 2002. Rural health care providers in the United States. *Journal of Rural Health* 18(S):211–232.

Hartley D, Bird D, Dempsey P. 1999. Rural mental health and substance abuse. In: Ricketts TC, ed. *Rural Health in the United States.* New York: Oxford University Press. Pp. 159–178.

Hartley D, Hart V, Hanrahan N, Loux S. 2004. *Are Advanced Practice Psychiatric Nurses a Solution to Rural Mental Health Workforce Shortages.* Portland, ME: Maine Rural Health Research Center, University of Southern Maine.

Hooker R, Berline LE. 2002. Trends in the supply of physician assistants and nurse practitioners in the United States. *Health Affairs* 21(5):164–181.

Horgan C, Levine H. 1998. The substance abuse treatment system: What does it look like and whom does it serve? In: Lamb S, Greenlick MR, McCarty D, eds. *Bridging the Gap Between Practice and Research: Forging Partnerships with Community-Based Drug and Alcohol Treatment.* Washington, DC: National Academy Press.

HRSA (Health Resources and Services Administration). 2000. *The Pharmacist Workforce: A Study of the Supply and Demand for Pharmacists.* Washington, DC: U.S. Department of Health and Human Services.

HRSA. 2003. *Access to Emergency Medical Devices Grant Program.* [Online]. Available: http://www.apcointl.org/frequency/DEPARTMENTOFHEALTHANDHUMAN SERVICES.htm [accessed June 2, 2004].

HRSA. 2004. *HRSA Issue Brief: The New Medicare Rural Hospital Flexibility Program.* [Online]. Available: http://ruralhealth.hrsa.gov/pub/IssueBrief1.htm [accessed May 2004].

Hutchison L, Blakely C. 2003. Substance abuse-trends in rural areas: A literature review. In: Gamm L, Hutchison L, Dabney BD, Dorsey AM, eds. *Rural Healthy People 2010: A Companion Document to Healthy People 2010. Volume 2.* College Station, TX: Texas A&M University System Health Science Center, School of Rural Public Health, Southwest Rural Health Research Center.

IOM (Institute of Medicine). 1988. *The Future of Public Health.* Washington, DC: National Academy Press.

IOM. 1992. *Emerging Infections: Microbial Threats to Health.* Washington, DC: National Academy Press.

IOM. 1996. *Primary Care: America's Health in a New Era.* Washington, DC: National Academy Press.

IOM. 1997a. *America's Vital Interest in Global Health.* Washington, DC: National Academy Press.

IOM. 1997b. *Improving Health in the Community: A Role for Performance Monitoring.* Washington, DC: National Academy Press.

IOM. 2000. *America's Safety Net: Intact but Endangered.* Washington, DC: National Academy Press.

IOM. 2001. *Improving the Quality of Long Term Care.* Washington, DC: National Academy Press.

IOM. 2003. *The Future of the Public's Health in the 21st Century.* Washington, DC: The National Academies Press.

Ivey SL, Scheffler R, Zazzali JL. 1998. Supply dynamics of the mental health workforce: Implications for health policy. *Milbank Quarterly* 76(1):25–28.

Johnson R, Morris TF. 2000. *Stabilizing the Rural Public Health Infrastructure.* Washington, DC: National Advisory Committee on Rural Health and Human Services, U.S. Department of Health and Human Services.

Kessler RC, McGonagle KA, Zhao S, Nelson CB, Hughes M, Eschleman S, Wittchen HU, Kendler KS. 1994. Lifetime and 12-month prevalence of DSM-III-R psychiatric disorders in the United States: Results from the national comorbidity survey. *Archives of General Psychiatry* 51:8–19.

LaLonde M. 1975. *A New Perspective on the Health of Canadians.* Ottawa, Canada: Ministry of National Health and Welfare.

Lambert D, Agger MS. 1995. Access of rural AFDC Medicaid beneficiaries to mental health services. *Health Care Financing Review* 17(1):133–145.

Larson EH, Norris TE. 2003. Rural Demography and the Health Workforce: Interstate Comparisons. In: Larson EH, Johnson KE, Norris TE, Lishner DM, Rosenblatt RA, Hart LG, eds. *State of the Health Workforce in Rural America. Profiles and Comparisons.* Seattle, WA: WWAMI. Pp. 23–44.

Larson SL, Machlin S, Nixon A, Zodet M. 2003. *Urban/Rural Comparisons of Health Care Access, Use, and Expenses, 1998–2000 (Average Annual).* Washington, DC: Agency for Healthcare Research and Quality, U.S. Department of Health and Human Services.

MedPAC. 2001. *Report to the Congress: Medicare in Rural America.* Washington, DC: MedPAC.

MedPAC. 2004. *Report to Congress: Medicare Payment Policy.* Washington, DC: MedPAC.

Merwin E, Mauck A. 1995. Psychiatric nursing outcome research: The state of science. *Archives of Psychiatric Nursing* 9(6):311–331.

Mohatt DF, Mock J, Adams SJ, Shaw J. 2003. *Rural Mental Health WICHE West: Meeting Workforce Demands through Regional Partnership.* Paper presented at the meeting of the Frontier Mental Health Workshop Roundtable. Reno, NV: WICHE.

Mohr PE. 2003. *Survey of Critical Access-Affiliated Emergency Medical Service Providers.* Bethesda, MD: Project HOPE Walsh Center for Rural Health Analysis.

Moorhead JC, Gallery ME, Hirshkorn C, Barnaby DP, Barsan WG, Conrad LC, Dalsey WC, Fried M, Herman SH, Hogan P, Mannle TE, Packard DC, Perina DG, Pollack CV Jr, Rapp MT, Rorrie CC Jr, Schafermeyer RW. 2002. A study of the workforce in emergency medicine. *Annals of Emergency Medicine* 40(1):3–18.

Morrisey MA, Ohsfelt RL, Johnson V, Treat R. 1995. Rural emergency medical services: Patients, destinations, times, and services. *Journal of Rural Health* 11(4):286–294.

Moscovice I, Stensland J. 2002. Rural hospitals: Trends, challenges, and a future research and policy agenda analysis. *Journal of Rural Health* 18(S):197–210.

NACRHHS (National Advisory Committee on Rural Health and Human Services). 2000. *Rural Public Health: Issues and Considerations.* Washington, DC: U.S. Department of Health and Human Services.

Narrow WE, Rae DS, Robins LN, Regier DA. 2002. Revised prevalence estimates of mental disorders in the United States. *Archives of General Psychiatry* 59:115–123.

NCHS (National Center for Health Statistics). 2001. *Health, United States, 2001 with Urban and Rural Health Chartbook.* Washington, DC: U.S. Department of Health and Human Services.

NFCMH (New Freedom Commission on Mental Health). 2003. *Achieving the Promise: Transforming Mental Health Care in America.* [Online]. Available: http://www.mentalhealthcommission.gov/ [accessed June 9, 2004].

Nichols L. 2004. *Oral Health Partnership Leads to Cost-Effective Care.* [Online]. Available: http://www.nachc.com/HCW/Files/NACHC-CHF.pdf [accessed June 30, 2004].

North M. 2004. *CHC Faces Staffing Challenge for New Dental Clinic.* [Online]. Available: http://www.nachc.com/HCW/Files/NACHC-CHF.pdf [accessed June 30, 2004].

NRC (National Research Council). 2002. *Making the Nation Safer: The Role of Science and Technology in Countering Terrorism.* Washington, DC: The National Academies Press.

NRHA (National Rural Health Association). 2001a. *Policy Brief: Long-Term Care in Rural America*. [Online]. Available: http://www.nrharural.org/pagefile/issuepapers/ipaper21.html [accessed July 12, 2004].

NRHA. 2001b. *Oral Health in America: A Rural Perspective (A Companion to the Surgeon General's Report on Oral Health)*. Notes: A White Paper by the National Rural Health Association with funding by ORHP.

OAS (Office of Applied Studies). 2003. *The NHSDA Report: Substance Abuse or Dependence in Metropolitan and Non-Metropolitan Areas*. Rockville, MD: OAS.

ODP (Office for Domestic Preparedness). 2004 (May). *Support for the Emergency Medical Service Provided Through the Office for Domestic Preparedness*. Washington, DC: U.S. Department of Homeland Security.

ODPHP (Office of Disease Prevention and Health Promotion). 2000. *Healthy People 2010*. [Online]. Available: http://www.healthypeople.gov/ [accessed June 8, 2004].

Okwumabua JO, Baker FM, Wong SP, Pilgram BO. 1997. Characteristics of depressive symptoms in elderly urban and rural African Americans. *Journal of Gerontology: Medical Sciences* 52A:M241–M246.

OMB (Office of Management and Budget). 2000. *Standards for Defining Metropolitan and Micropolitan Statistical Areas*. [Online]. Available: http://www.census.gov/population/www/estimates/00-32997.pdf [accessed May 2003].

ORHP (Office of Rural Health Policy). 2002. *One Department Serving Rural America*. DHHS Rural Task Force, Washington, DC: U.S. Department of Health and Human Services.

OTA (Office of Technology Assessment). 1989. *Special Report: Rural Emergency Medical Services*. Washington, DC: U.S. Government Printing Office.

Phillips CD, Hawes C, Williams ML. 2003. *Nursing Homes in Rural and Urban Areas, 2000*. College Station, TX: Southwest Rural Health Research Center, Texas A&M University.

Phillips RL, Green LA. 2002. Making choices about the scope of family practice. *Journal of the American Board of Family Practice* 15(3):250–254.

Phillips RL Jr, Harper DC, Wakefield M, Green LA, Fryer GE Jr. 2002. Can nurse practitioners and physicians beat pariochialism into plowshares? *Health Affairs* 21(5):133–142.

Probst J, Samuels M, Hussey J, Berry D, Ricketts T. 1999. Economic impact of hospital closure on small rural counties, 1984 to 1988: Demonstration of a comparative analysis approach. *Journal of Rural Health* 15(4):375–390.

Rawlinson C, Crews P. 2003. Access to quality health services in rural areas—Emergency medical services: A literature review. In: Gamm L, Hutchison L, Dabney B, Dorsey A, eds. *Rural Healthy People 2010. Access to Quality Health Services in Rural Areas*. College Station, TX: Southwest Rural Health Research Center, Texas A&M University. Pp. 77–81.

Regier DA, Narrow WE, Rae DS, Manderscheid RW, Locke BZ, Goodwin FK. 1993. The de facto U.S. mental and addictive disorders service system: Epidemiologic catchment area prospective 1-year prevalence rates of disorders and services. *Archives of General Psychiatry* 50:85–94.

Ricketts TC. 1999. *Rural Health in the United States*. New York: Oxford University Press.

Rosenblatt R. 2002. Quality of care in the rural context: A proposed research agenda. *Journal of Rural Health* 18(S):176–185.

Rosenthal MB, Zaslavsky AM, Newhouse JP. 2003. *The Geographic Distribution of Physician Revisited.* Boston, MA: Harvard School of Public Health, Harvard University.

Rost K, Fortney J, Fischer E, Smith J. 2002. Use, quality, and outcomes of care for mental health: The rural perspective. *Medical Care Research and Review* 59(3):231–265.

SAMHSA (Substance Abuse and Mental Health Services Administration). 2003. *Alcohol and Drug Services Study (ADSS): The National Substance Abuse Treatment System: Facilities, Clients, Services, and Staffing.* Rockville, MD: SAMHSA, OAS.

Shelton DA, Merwin EI, Fox JC. 1995. Implications of health care reform for rural mental health services. *Administration and Policy in Mental Health* 23:59–69.

Stensland J, Davidson G, Moscovice I. 2004. *The Financial Benefits of Critical Access Hospital Conversion for FY 1999 and FY 2000 Converters.* Minneapolis, MN: Rural Health Research Center, University of Minnesota.

Stillner V, Kraus RF, Leukefeld CG, Hardenbergh D. 1999. Drug use in very rural Alaska villages. *Substance Use and Misuse* 34(4–5):579–593.

USDHHS (U.S. Department of Health and Human Services). 2000. *Healthy People 2010: Understanding and Improving Health.* Washington, DC: U.S. Department of Health and Human Services.

USDOT (U.S. Department of Transportation). 1998. *Emergency Medical Services: Agenda for the Future.* Washington, DC: U.S. Department of Transportation.

USPHS (U.S. Public Health Service). 1999. *Mental Health: A Report of the Surgeon General.* Washington, DC: U.S. Department of Health and Human Services.

USPHS. 2000. *Oral Health in America: A Report of the Surgeon General.* Washington, DC: U.S. Department of Health and Human Services.

Wagenfeld MO, Murray JD, Mohatt DF, DeBruyn JC. 1994. *Mental Health and Rural America: 1980–1993. An Overview and Annotated Bibliography.* ORHP, U.S. DHHS NIH Pub. No. 94-3500:1–116.

WHA (Wisconsin Hospital Association). 2004. *Who Will Care for Our Patients? Wisconsin Takes Action to Fight a Growing Physician Shortage.* Madison, WI: Task Force on Wisconsin's Future Physician Workforce.

Williams D. 2003. *Remarks to the National Mental Health Association. HRSA Newsroom.* [Online]. Available: http://newsroom.hrsa.gov/speeches/2003speeches/NMHA.htm [accessed December 2003].

Williams JM, Ehrlich PF, Prescott JE. 2001. Emergency medical care in rural America. *Annals of Emergency Medicine* 38(3):323–327.

Wolff TL, Dewar J, Tudiver F. 2001. Chapter 12: Rural mental health. In: *Textbook of Rural Medicine.* New York: McGraw-Hill Medical Publishing Division. Pp. 181–194.

Index